Praise for
Hernzebekana! Her Language of Love

This book is the essence of the tragedy and triumph of people with brain injury. Becki's story takes you back to the first inkling of an "episode" as a sixth grader that might have been the start of her first AVM aneurysm 13 years later. Now, almost 60 years afterwards, Becki, along with her family and friends, describes her aphasia and stroke-strewn journey while still thriving through her joy-filled life in the face of it all with humor and grace.

—Thomas G. Broussard, Jr., Ph.D.,
three-time stroke survivor, president & founder, Aphasia Nation, Inc.
And Johnny Appleseed of Aphasia Awareness

"Hernzebekana: Her Language of Love," written by Rebecca Lawton and Dawn Rosewitz, is a memoir about a multiple-stroke survivor who has aphasia. It takes us through her life and struggles after surviving multiple strokes. When words don't work, what are we left with? The memoir gives us some answers to those questions, as well as the everyday struggles that aphasic patients go through. The book is told from several different perspectives, including the actual patient and her family. When words didn't work, one word worked really well – "Hernzebekana."
...This memoir keeps the reader engaged and gives a different perspective than most books I've read. Becki is truly an inspiration for everyone. This memoir should be read by all medical personnel who have any interaction with stroke survivors, so they have a better understanding of the foreign lands that these survivors are navigating.

—Amber Koll PA-C, MPAS, EMT-P
Internal Medicine

Hernzebekana!

Her Language of Love

Hernzebekana!

Her Language of Love

When Words Fail:
The Memoir of a Multiple-Stroke Survivor with Aphasia

Rebecca Lawton
Dawn Rosewitz

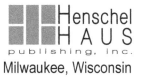

Henschel
HAUS
publishing, inc.
Milwaukee, Wisconsin

Published by HenschelHAUS Publishing, Inc.
Milwaukee, Wisconsin
www.henschelHAUSbooks.com

ISBN: 978159598-928-4
E-ISBN: 978159598-929-1
LCCN: 2022944758

Printed in the United States of America.

Cover photo by Dawn Rosewitz

Dedications & Acknowledgments

Becki

So many people have been important parts of my support group in so many ways during my journey as a stroke survivor— including some who are no longer with us. I could write an entire book (with Dawn's assistance, of course!) just listing and thanking you. But you all know who you are. I extend a special thanks to Avery, who reviewed the book early on and helped with PowerPoint presentations, and to my sister Gretch who provided material for the book.

Specifically, however, I want to thank Dawn with all my heart for having painstakingly spent so many long hours listening to what I had to say and then putting it in words on paper. I am forever indebted to you and thankful for what you have done for me. And Dawn and I both extend our special acknowledgment and thank you to Judith Gwinn Adrian, who did the final editorial review and helped facilitate our path to publication of the book. The passion and compassion that Judith and our publisher, Kira Henschel, had for our story is very much appreciated and has been very serendipitous to get us to this point after so many years. And thank you, Larry Cockerel, for bringing them to us.

I also want to thank the wonderful speech therapists who have been in my life: Becky, Kathy, Mary, Linda, Necia, Dana, Barbara, and, of course, my daughter Aimee. And I am especially indebted to my two neurosurgeons, who created the dents in my head that my grandchildren love to rub!

I dedicate this book to Denny: my teacher, my coach, my love.

I also dedicate it to my parents, Cal and Velda, who are now with the Lord; my two beautiful daughters—Aimee and Abie—and the eight wonderful grandchildren I am lucky enough to enjoy having in my life: Karis, Otto, Sophie, Kannon, Ainsley, Adele, Krewe, and Kliegh.

DAWN

When I first met Becki, I was starting a new job as a special education teacher at Cedarburg High School, in Wisconsin. My first impression? She was like a stand-up comedian, always ready with a joke or song (continuously off-key). But there wasn't a person in the school who didn't know and appreciate Becki's humor and unique perspective on life. Her special talent, though, was reaching out to the most difficult students. She generated such a love for them; they always knew they could come to her with their problems and she would do her best to help them. She was quick with a hug or her infamous humor.

I loved working with Becki. So, when she asked me to write her story—one I hadn't totally understood yet—I said yes. After two years of discussion, we finally put her story into words, working together to pull all the fragmented pieces together.

Becki, it is a blessing to know you, and I thank God you're still with us to tell your story. I devote this book to every person who has ever struggled with a disability and found the strength to not only live with it, but to transcend it, as Becki has. Thank you, Becki and Denny, for entrusting me with your story!

To my amazing parents, Harold and Marge, with love and gratitude. Words cannot express what a blessing you both are. Sorry for all the gray hairs and sleepless nights (but the other kids were worse, except for Tracey who got away with more because she was sneakier than the rest). To Anna, Mike, and Kayla, I'm blessed to be a part of your life. To Carol and Kim, my second mom and sister, I treasure you both. To Ken, for bringing love and humor to my second chapter along with Connor, Shayla and the rest of your wonderfully crazy family. And to the rest of my family, especially Nicky, Roy, Steve, Jenny, Tracey, Mike, Robin, Steve, Gina and Dixon, even though some of you drove me crazy half my life. You know who you are…

TABLE OF CONTENTS

FOREWORD

THE FIRST TIME I ENCOUNTERED A STROKE victim, I was in the 5th grade. My class had "adopted" grandparents from the local nursing home and in spring, we had an opportunity visit with them. The entire year I watched as my classmates received letters from their "adopted grandparent" and I thought, "Why isn't Basil writing back to me?"

I couldn't fully comprehend at the time that because of his stroke he wasn't able to write to me. When I met him on that beautiful spring day, my teacher smiled at me and said, "I knew you would be able to take on this challenge." His eyes sparkled as a crooked smile came across his face. I approached him and presented the artwork I had created as a gift. He mumbled something I couldn't understand. He was in there; I knew it.

Thus began the journey of my desire to help those who struggled to communicate. I didn't know what aphasia was, but I did know it must be the most frustrating thing and I wanted to help.

Hernzebekana! Her Language of Love captures the struggles and victories of the lifetime of Rebecca (Becki), a multiple stroke victim living with the effects of aphasia. The style and detail presented in this memoir keeps the reader engaged and provides perspective that many overlook. Those living with aphasia and the residual effects of a stroke are navigating a foreign world. Becki's story invites the reader to see this world, and walk a few steps in the shoes of an aphasic. Her courage and strength, coupled with a phenomenal sense of humor and faith, is a beacon of inspiration for all.

Melissa Kaiser, MS, CCC-SLP
is a Speech and Language Pathologist with over 30 years of experience working in communication disorders. She completed an internship at the Milwaukee VA Hospital, specifically working with stroke victims. She then worked at Cedar Haven Rehabilitation Agency before transitioning to the high school setting. She shares Becki's passion for working with youth and adding humor to connect with others.

INTRODUCTION

IN THE FALL OF 1963, WHILE in 6th grade, Becki (Miller) Lawton experienced a two-week episode of lost speech and headaches, spending ten days in the hospital. The episode was not formally diagnosed at the time, but was thought to possibly be encephalitis. Although Becki's school performance did change somewhat after that episode, with studying for tests and memory work becoming more difficult, she completed high school with good grades and went on to receive a B.A. degree in English from Valparaiso University in 1974.

On February 1, 1976, at the age of 24, three months after giving birth to her first daughter, Aimee, and two weeks after having had gallbladder surgery, Becki suffered a severe hemorrhagic stroke related to the rupture of an arteriovenous malformation (AVM), an aneurysm of blood vessels that had been growing on the left side of her brain since birth.

Although receiving an ominous prognosis by doctors at the time, after one month in intensive care and a little more than two months total in the hospital, Becki began her road to recovery, striving to lead as normal a life as possible with her permanent residual aphasia, an impairment of verbal and reading expression and comprehension.

Becki's recovery included giving birth to her second daughter, Abie, in 1980, numerous sessions with several speech therapists, and going through vocational rehabilitation. After the disappointment of being told her employment expectations were

1

unreasonable, she set out on her own to find a job that resulted in a 13-year career as a special education paraprofessional.

On October 12, 1998, after always thinking the chance for recurrence of a similar stroke was slim, Becki suffered another, less severe, hemorrhagic stroke related to the same AVM. Her road to recovery continued, but with a new detour. After suffering the strokes from the AVM in 1976 and 1998, Becki's family and doctors surmised that the two-week episode of lost speech and headaches in 6th grade also was likely a hemorrhagic stroke due to the same AVM.

In *Hernzebekana! Her Language of Love*, Becki and co-author, Dawn Rosewitz, tell Becki's story of her early years as a young, multiple stroke survivor. The story starts briefly with the day of her 1998 stroke, then transitions back to the period from the first severe stroke in 1976 through the hospitalization for the 1998 stroke.

A brief epilogue provides a synopsis of Becki's recovery, challenges, and joys since her 1998 stroke. These first-person recollections from Becki, family members, and friends provide the unique perspectives of those who have experienced and are impacted by strokes and aphasia.

And *hernzebekana*? What? Don't you know the word? Well, when words fail Becki, which happens on occasion, *hernzebekana* (pronounced hern-ze-ba-ka-na, emphasis on the first syllable) is one word she can always say. It is her word. It is her family's word. They all know *hernzebekana*! It is the keystone to her language of love.

PREFACE

QUITE FRANKLY, I WAS NOT REALLY that excited when Becki first told me she was going to write a book about her stroke and aphasia experiences, especially when she said the format would be such that my personal thoughts would be portrayed. I soon realized that writing this book was important for Becki and could perhaps also help other stroke victims and their families. Though we never really thought our lives were more unique or challenging than those of others, having survived three strokes and living with aphasia for 46 years, and being the spouse of an aphasic stroke survivor for almost five decades (1976–2022), has provided us with a unique experience, and also many blessings.

I think the biggest message Becki wants to tell by both her book and in her daily life is that people with aphasia are not stupid; they just have short circuits in their communication network, which are not their fault. Becki's brain trauma events have resulted in her having a somewhat unique personality that some people can relate to and appreciate, while others, quite frankly, are taken aback and don't quite know what to think. Many people who meet Becki, and some who have known her for some time, may not be able to tell she has a disability. Most people, likely including myself at times, do not fully understand how difficult it is for Becki to do certain things, especially trying to follow a fast or complicated conversation, or just making her feet and arms work in sequence when going for a walk. Becki has learned to compensate for her disabilities through her 46 years of practice.

A defining moment for Becki on her road to recovery was when she received evaluation and training through a vocational rehabilitation program. A Ph.D. psychologist evaluated her toward the end of the program and suggested she was not employable and should consider applying for Social Security Insurance Disability benefits. That really ticked Becki off. After struggling in her first couple job placements, because people did not truly understand the disabilities of a person with aphasia, she found a job on her own as a special education paraprofessional— a job for which she had a unique sense of understanding and compassion. Although this was not what she envisioned after graduating from college with a degree in English and a desire to pursue a law degree, God apparently had a different plan for Becki. She continued working in special education for 13 years.

Becki's life experiences have also touched and guided the lives of other people. When we lived in Nebraska, a young lady from our church youth group pursued a career in speech pathology, partly due to Becki's suggestion and encouragement to give it a try. Our oldest daughter, Aimee, also became a speech pathologist, having been influenced by the daily challenges she witnessed her mother face.

Although part of Becki's wanting to tell her story is to help other aphasic stroke survivors and their families, this can be a double-edged sword. We have had several opportunities to interact with families of stroke patients. In some cases, the family members looked at Becki's recovery and had unrealistic expectations for their family member's recovery. In other cases, we could sense the family members thinking, "Oh my God! Is this the best it is going to get?"

Every brain trauma situation is different, and the nature and degree of physical or communication disability varies significantly, so we suggest being careful not to judge expected outcomes for your loved ones based on those of others.

Preface

We also have found that many, even in the medical professions, do not always understand the specific individual challenges of a person with aphasia. Over the years, we have had many wonderful doctors and other medical professionals. We are very grateful for them. There have also been some experiences where they did not seem to understand that the mind of an aphasic works differently. We learned that family members can provide valuable insights to the medical professionals and be important advocates for their loved ones.

I want to especially express my appreciation to co-author Dawn Rosewitz. Becki verbally provided and recorded thoughts on tape for Dawn, who put them on paper, which was not always an easy task. Dawn and Becki met numerous times over the course of two summers and during a school year, at coffee shops, parks, and our respective homes. Recollecting experiences and events from 25 to 45 years ago also provided challenges, although many of the experiences seemed like they occurred just yesterday. Dawn's diligence and dedication in helping re-create Becki's story is almost a journey in itself. Although it has been several years since Becki and Dawn completed the first draft of the book, getting to this point of publication now is awesome!

We also want to emphasize that our faith and trust in God has provided us the strength to meet the daily challenges. Our faith and the spiritual support of our families and friends has been a constant blessing.

Dennis (Denny) Lawton
(Becki's Husband)

CHAPTER 1

NOT AGAIN

OCTOBER 1998: A GOOD WEEKEND THAT ENDS IN PAIN
(Flash Forward)

BECKI

It's going to be such a good weekend. The energy in the halls and classrooms as teenagers prepare for the homecoming activities is contagious. After school, I meet our new special education teacher, Dawn, for the parade downtown. Then I head back home to pick up my husband, Denny, for the football game. Once we find a spot on the bleachers, we are soon surrounded by a screaming mass of teenagers and parents for the big homecoming football game. This year we play the Knights, a tough team, but I am sure we'll beat them. Now, some people might think the noise and pounding feet would get tiresome, but I find it invigorating. The excitement of a new school year fills the stadium, and all I can think about is the new bunch of students I started working with this year. In my overexuberance, I shout out to a familiar face,

"Hey, teenager, you're in trouble now!" Knowing that I love to tease, the student rolls his eyes and grins back at me.

"Yeah, right, Mrs. Lawton. I didn't do nothin'."

"Okay, teenager," I say in a mock threatening voice, "don't talk smart or I'll haul your butt into Principal Rieger's office."

Of course, the student knows I am all talk and turns back to his friends, laughing. Then I look for my next teenage target, and since I know so many of the students, I spend most of the football game exchanging friendly fire with them. This is my way of interacting and reaching the students. I had made many a friend with students in the special education program because I always incorporate humor into our conversations along with, of course, a big dose of respect for their uniquenesses as young adults.

* * *

When we go to bed Sunday night, Denny says, "It's been a good weekend," and it truly has.

I feel blessed to be working in the high school special education program, blessed by my family, and proud of my two beautiful daughters, Aimee and Abie. Everything in my world seems perfect. I cuddle up next to Denny and close my eyes.

As I'm just starting to fall asleep, a stabbing pain runs through the back of my head. "Ooh," I groan and jerk backward.

Denny rolls over and faces me. "You okay?"

"Yeah," I say, and I'm not lying, because the pain disappears as quickly as it comes. "Just a little twinge."

In a few hours though, the pain is back and unrelenting. It feels like someone's probing inside my brain. Denny gives me Tylenol, but it doesn't ease the pain. If anything, it's worse. Maybe if I reposition myself, it'll stop. I roll over onto my stomach and cover the back of my head with both hands, trying to stop the threat creeping through my brain. Then I feel something shift, and I panic.

The invisible monster is back!

The pressure continues to build on the left side of my head. It's like déjà vu, and although now I'm forty-six, I feel like that twenty-four-year-old woman again, lying in my bed wondering when this headache will end. This time, though, I'm not only wondering when it will end, but how.

It's strange the things you remember when something life-altering happens to you. You'd think I would remember the pain of that first stroke in February 1976, but I don't, even though I am told I complained of a bad headache. I can recall looking out my window on that cold February morning and seeing the shimmering icicles hanging precariously from the tree branches, translucent under the moon and dripping slowly to the frosted earth. But mostly, I remember how that one day in 1976 changed my whole life, for that headache wasn't merely a headache. It was an aneurysm that ruptured and damaged the left side of my brain, causing me to quickly fall into a coma. When I came out of the coma, I had to fight for every lost memory and every lost word. I can't help worrying now. I can't bear to go through that again.

I can't go through this again.
Now, once again the steady pounding inside my head shatters the quiet of an early morning, and I cling to the reassurance of Denny's rhythmic soft breaths against my cheek. Abie is sleeping like a baby, although now a young lady, a senior in high school.

"Denny," I say and nudge him slightly. "Can you get me some water?"

He nods sleepily and refills the water glass next to me.

Please God, I beg, not again. I make up all kinds of excuses. I have a new job. I'm too old to go through this again. We're finally taking that romantic trip to San Francisco we've dreamed about. Abie still needs me at home, etc,, etc.

Still the pounding continues. I can't believe, after twenty-two years, it is happening again.

Then the realization that this isn't going to go away sinks in. I call out to Denny, barely audible, choking on each word. "Denny, I'm doing it again," like I have any control over it. I know I have none.

I hear the glass in Denny's hand shatter on the bathroom floor and realize I won't be going to work today.

I know I have to be brave. There must be another blood vessel breaking open somewhere inside my head, just like before. I bury my face in the pillow and close my eyes tightly, trying to keep myself together, trying to stay in control. I know I have to muster the courage to go through this again.

CHAPTER 2

MEMORIES OF THREE BUSY MONTHS

NOVEMBER 1975 TO JANUARY 1976
AIMEE IS BORN

BECKI

I STEP, OR SHOULD I SAY WADDLE, into the doctor's office. According to earlier tests, I should be giving birth tomorrow and this is just my 24-hour pre-labor checkup.

"Looks like you're dilated three centimeters now," Dr. Pavlock tells me. "How do you feel?"

I toss that one around in my head. Let's see. *How do I feel?* I feel like I've got a pair of ten-pound bowling balls in my belly, my legs look like sausages, and my chin has slid down into my neck. But I don't tell him that. Instead, I say, "Ready to deliver."

Dr. Pavlock nods and checks my blood pressure. "Your blood pressure is way up." He raises his eyebrows, which makes waves of wrinkles appear on his forehead. He taps his pen for a moment as he runs an idea through his head.

"I think you've been pregnant long enough, and since you're ready, let's not wait until tomorrow. Let's get things going now and introduce you to your baby. Why don't you go get Denny and meet me at the hospital?"

Even with my protruding belly, there's still room for butterflies in there.

After making plans with Dr. Pavlock, I leave in search of Denny on campus. I think I know where he is. It's about 11a.m., so he should be heading to the student union cafeteria for lunch. I know I'll have to catch him before he heads off to the library to work on his thesis. In my condition, it will take me ages to find him in there. Luckily, I catch him just before he leaves for lunch.

Denny sees the excitement on my face then looks at my belly. "Everything okay?"

"Kinda'," I grin. "We have to go have a baby now."

Denny stares at me blankly. "Today?"

I wrap my arm around his. "Yes, today."

There's a long pause before Denny asks, "Do I have time for a sandwich?"

I look at him in disbelief. I'm about to have a baby and he wants to get a sandwich!

"Fine." I say, gritting my teeth. "But only one," and as an afterthought I add, "with no pickles on it." If I have to suffer watching him eat it, he can suffer without the pickles.

* * *

"One more push, Becki," says Dr. Pavlock.

"That's what you said last time," I groan and muster the rest of my energy for what should, hopefully, be the last push. Suddenly there's a loud cry and a shuffling around me.

"We've got a baby girl, Bec," Denny tells me. He brings her closer so I can get a better look. She wriggles and lets out a scream.

"Just like her mother," Denny jokes.

"Ha, ha," I tell him. "Let's hope she looks like me too." Right now, it's hard to tell who she looks like, although luckily, she doesn't have a beard like Denny. She's all pink and blotchy. I do know one thing for sure (and I don't think I'm biased), she's the most beautiful baby I've ever seen. "Aimee," I whisper, content, and lie back down.

LOTS GOING ON

BECKI

Aimee gets to go to her first basketball game, about a week after coming home, watching Denny play on our church's basketball team. I think some of the other ladies question us taking her out so early, but we think she should start experiencing the world as early as possible.

Later in November, we take Aimee with us to Elgin, Illinois, to watch her Uncle Jim get married to her new Aunt Becky, and meet lots of the other Miller and Van Eman family members.

Then we are back in Elgin again in early December for Aimee's baptism at Good Shepherd Lutheran Church, where I was baptized and Denny and I were married.

We spend Aimee's first Christmas in Elgin, then we travel to visit with Denny's family in Richland Center, Wisconsin. After enjoying a Friday night fish fry in Richland Center, I end up in the emergency room with a terrible pain in my side. We don't know if it is due to the fish fry or something else.

Denny doesn't have to go back to school until mid-January. After our visit with Denny's parents, we go back to Elgin so Mom can take us all down to Petersburg, Illinois, to introduce Aimee to her Great-grandma Van Eman. Again, the first night at Grandma Van's, my night's sleep is interrupted by that same terrible pain in my side.

Mom, being the insightful nurse that she is, piles us into the car in the middle of the night and we head back to Elgin. Before I know it, I am in a hospital bed recovering from gallbladder surgery.

After some initial recovery from surgery, we head back to Milwaukee, looking forward to a less busy and less eventful start to our life with Aimee.

CHAPTER 3

The First Big Boom

FEBRUARY 1, 1976 – PAIN, THEN NOTHING

BECKI

IT'S EARLY SUNDAY MORNING AND for once the house is quiet. Aimee is due for her bottle soon and since sleep seems to be a luxury these days, I decide to indulge a little longer. I am moving a little slower since having my gallbladder removed about two weeks ago, but Denny's sister, Sandy, is staying with us this weekend to help.

The past few months have been a whirlwind for me, what with giving birth to Aimee three months ago, Jim and Becky's wedding, the baptism, and then the gallbladder surgery. Denny heads out to Texas tomorrow morning for a job interview with a major oil company. I hear that big things happen in threes. I have a feeling moving will be next, and what could the third event awaiting us be?

Last night, Sandy stayed with Aimee so that Denny and I could go out and meet some friends at the bowling alley. My head was a bit stuffed up, so we stopped off at a gas station and picked up some nose spray. I wasn't quite up to bowling yet because of my gallbladder surgery, but that didn't stop me from thoroughly enjoying the evening. After we got home, I quickly crawled into bed and fell fast asleep.

In the early morning hours, I'm awakened by what feels like a head cold, making me think my brain will explode at any moment. I make sure to get up slowly and sit for a minute. Luckily, Aimee's not crying to be fed yet. Maybe if I sit up, the stuffiness will drain out and give me some relief. But as I lean forward, a sharp pain knocks me back down. I wince and grab my head. Bad idea. I lie back down. My arm feels heavy as I try to reach for Denny across the bed.

"Can you get me an aspirin?"

"Sure," he says, "Is it a bad one?"

"Not too bad," I lie and bury my head deeper into the pillow. "Just need an aspirin."

Something strange is happening. Spots of color—red, orange, blue—begin exploding in my head like fireworks. Then there is nothing.

DENNY

"Becki," is all I can say as I try to control her convulsions.

Don't panic, I tell myself over and over, but I can't stop my heart from pounding in my throat. As if on automatic pilot, I call for an ambulance.

"My wife's having a seizure," I explain, trying to stay calm.

The operator asks all kinds of questions. "Is she getting any air? What was she doing before it happened? How long was the last seizure?"

I try to keep focused. "Sleeping. Two minutes." More questions. I wonder where the ambulance is. "Please just send someone."

"We have an ambulance on the way, sir. It should be there any second now."

I drop the phone as Becki goes into another seizure. Her whole body stiffens. Then her head arches back and her arms flail violently against the bed. "It'll be okay, Bec," I try to reassure her, but I don't know if she can even hear me.

In the next room, Aimee begins to stir. It's time for her morning bottle, but I need to be with Bec. Sandy is in the other room and hears all the commotion. She comes to check on us. I don't need to say much because she can quickly see that something is terribly wrong.

"The ambulance is on the way," I tell her.

"What should I do?"

"Just watch Aimee, okay?"

Sandy nods. "Okay."

I turn back to Bec. Thing is, I'm not sure what needs to be done next. I'm a scientist. I should know what to do, but I don't. I can only wait...

One more strong seizure hits Becki. It's another long minute before it ends. Then her body relaxes and she begins to breathe again. I touch her face and arms. Her skin is pale and clammy. She's never looked so fragile before. I make sure she doesn't hurt herself. When I pull the blanket back, I notice a wet spot forming around her thighs—the result of the last seizure—and then I think about how embarrassed she'd be if anyone saw her in soiled clothes. I can't let her go to the hospital like that. My jeans are too big for her, but easy to get on. Then I hear the sirens. I take a deep breath. I have to remind myself to do that.

The paramedics check Bec's vitals and slowly lift her onto the gurney, making sure to keep her body straight and immobilizing her head.

"She's unconscious," they tell me.

* * *

Once we get to the emergency room, Becki is given one test after another. Blood tests followed by a spinal tap, and then more questions. "Is she allergic to anything?"

"No."

"Did she take any drugs before the seizure?"

"Only nose spray and aspirin."

The doctor looks at me with what feels like disbelief.

"Was your wife taking any other drugs?" he repeats. Looking at me like I'm a hippie from the seventies, he's already formed an opinion and assumed Bec has had a drug overdose.

"No," I respond defensively. "She doesn't do drugs. She had the start of a cold last night and took nose spray and aspirin. Before she had the seizure, she mentioned that her head hurt really bad. That's it."

The doctor is looking at something on his clipboard and rolling his lips between his teeth as if he's checking his words very carefully before he continues. Then he takes off his glasses and gives me a sympathetic look. "Mr. Lawton, are you sure your wife hasn't tried any other drugs? We need to know everything if we're going to help her. The severity of her seizures and her condition at the moment suggest to us that drugs may have been involved."

I can feel the heat rise to my face. We're wasting time with these questions. I struggle to keep my voice calm. "No, she has NOT taken drugs."

The doctor is about to speak again, but seeing the look on my face, thinks better of it and stops himself. Instead, he excuses himself to check on the results of her spinal tap. "I'll be right back."

Again, I'm left to my own thoughts while I wait for the results. To complete the spinal tap, the doctors threaded a needle into Becki's spine and withdrew some of the fluids. If there's blood in the fluid, there's a leak somewhere. Then they'll thread a tube through Becki's veins up to her brain to get a look at what's going on inside her head. Those pictures will then help them pinpoint exactly where Becki is bleeding and where they need to go in.

When another doctor returns, he has the results of Becki's tests. There are no more questions about drugs.

"They found blood in her spinal column. The neurosurgeon, Dr. Becker, thinks she may have a broken blood vessel somewhere, but we need to do an angiogram to get a better look." There is urgency in his voice. "If she is bleeding, we need to get in there fast and repair as much of the damage as we can." Then with some hesitation he asks, "Was she having headaches?"

"Yes," I tell him.

"You should've told us that sooner."

"I DID." That was the first thing I told them, but they probably saw my long hair and beard and drugs registered in their brains first. "I told the first doctor that," I explained, "but he didn't listen."

The doctor fidgets with his pen a moment. "Oh," he says. "We'll do all we can. Under the circumstances, I think we may need to get her into surgery immediately." Dr. Becker will look at this information then come and talk with you. I nod, and then he leaves.

While Becki is having the angiogram, her parents, Cal and Velda, arrive at the hospital. Afterwards, Dr. Becker and his partner, Dr. Uttech, stop to talk to us. They tell us a vessel has broken open on the left side of her brain and is leaking blood into the brain cavity. She's already been prepped for surgery. The left side of her head has been shaved where they will perform the operation.

As they are about to wheel her to an operating room, we walk beside her to the entrance and I squeeze her hand. She doesn't squeeze back, but I pray she knows I'm with her. Then she disappears behind the swinging doors.

The next few hours are pure hell. The staff is very good about keeping us updated on her progress. "They found a large malformed artery and hematoma (blood clot) on the left side of her brain which they're removing now. She's doing okay."

One of the doctors comes in with more good news. "She's made it through surgery. They've cleaned the area and closed it up. She'll be going to the post-op room overnight and they will continue to monitor her progress."

Medical records for February 1, 1976, summarize the events of the day:

The patient has been considered in good health until this morning on arising, she experienced a headache, became unresponsive and had convulsive seizures. The patient was admitted to the emergency room in extreme convulsing, valium anti-convulsant program was instituted, and the seizures were controlled...The patient remained unresponsive with minimally reactive pupils...

Respirations had never ceased but were increased in the course of the seizuring, as was the blood pressure. The patient was placed on emergency medical supportive measures and steroid therapy given...The patient has shown little response to the steroid therapy ...

Neurologically, the patient's state remained unchanged, she is in deep coma, myotic equal pupils, optic discs flat, neck rigid, eyes divergent, ...I have discussed with the family consideration that the hemorrhage may relate to arteriovenous malformation or statistically more likely, an aneurysm, though I am concerned of the former in view of seizure pattern though the seizures were non-focal. The need today for angiographic survey to be carried out to further define the intracranial status, rule out/identify a bleeding point, if possible, rule out intracerebral hematoma, and/or hydrocephalus.

The angiogram taken on that day reflected the doctor's concerns:

Impression: Obvious AV malformation in left posterior parietal area, fed by left posterior parietal and anterior carotid arteries. Significant hydrocephalus (fluid on the brain).

The doctors tell us that Becki is suffering from a ruptured cerebral aneurysm of an arteriovenous malformation (AVM). In layman's terms, Becki had a clump of blood vessels growing on the side of her brain that weren't supposed to be there. This morning, one of those vessels broke open. The clump, or malformation, had been there since birth but had gone undetected until today. For the most part, the vessels hadn't caused any problems until the aneurysm, a vessel that became swollen, broke open, and bled into other parts of her brain, causing the severe headache and seizures.

And that's when it really hits me. I almost lost her today. And I have no idea where we go from here!

GRETCH (BECKI'S SISTER)

Sunday, February 1, 1976, starts out like many other Sundays.

As my husband and I get ready for church, the snow falls hard and fast. I am preoccupied with thoughts of canceling the children's choir for services this morning due to the snow. Later, I am glad I had not, for the song they sang has been a bittersweet reminder of my much-needed faith.

Returning from communion, an usher stops and gives me a message to call my parents' home immediately. My mom tells me that my brother-in-law, Denny, called to tell them of my sister, Becki's, serious and life-threatening brain bleed. We are in shock. This doesn't happen to regular everyday people. This doesn't happen to people we love and cherish. This doesn't happen to my 24-year-old sister with a three-month-old baby and a husband in graduate school.

We rush to Milwaukee. Becki may not live through the day. As we leave the church to pack our bags, the snow becomes a serious problem. To our dismay, we discover roads are closed, and there's no way we can leave Rochelle for the two-and-a-half-hour drive to Milwaukee.

Finally, several hours later, the roads are plowed and we can leave.

Once we get to the hospital, we find my parents and Denny waiting outside the intensive care unit. Becki is in surgery. We learn that throughout the course of the afternoon, the bleeding had stopped, several tests have been given, and she's been diagnosed as having a massive hemorrhage of an AV malformation on the left side of her brain.

The First Big Boom

The surgery takes forever. One doctor gives us dim hope for her survival. On a scale of one to five, with five being death, Becki is given a four going into surgery. At nearly 1 a.m., Becki's neurosurgeon finds us to explain that Becki is miraculously still alive.

That's what matters most. She survived surgery. Whether or not she makes it through the night remains to be seen. Her doctor doesn't give us much hope for her surviving longer than a few days. She's suffered too much trauma. If she does live, he explains she could be in a coma for a long time. Then, if she survives the coma, she could come out a vegetable: blind, deaf, unemotional, and speechless.

After our talk with the doctor, we walk into the intensive care unit and see Becki for the first time. I swear it is someone else lying there. Her face is swollen and her head is covered with thick bandages. She is on life support and hooked up to a mass of wires and monitors. She is so still. I close my eyes and imagine the way she must've been just hours before, probably laughing and sharing stories with her friends. I open my eyes and press my face against Becki's hand.

No response.

Somehow, we all manage to get back to Denny and Becki's apartment to rest, but by 6 a.m., we are back at the hospital waiting for some sign of life from Becki. We sit and watch her. We stand and watch her. Then, when we can't take it any longer, we pace up and down the corridor, stopping only to look out the window at the icy Lake Michigan waters rolling forward and then slamming into the rocks. That beautiful sight fills me with such overwhelming sadness that I have to turn away.

Mom and Dad are mesmerized, though. More than once I find them staring out that window. Just staring. Mom is so entranced she seems to be off in another world, then suddenly acknowledges me with tears in her eyes. "How come I was so blessed for this long?" she asks.

"She's gonna' pull through, Mom."

Mom smiles weakly, then turns away, back to the window. I join my parents and watch the foam-capped waves stretch into the foggy horizon. We stay there for hours, praying for a miracle, waiting for Becki to wake up.

FLASHBACK TO 1963, SIXTH GRADE (STROKE #1?)

BECKI

Everything's surreal. The walls are moving. People's faces are a blur. I'm back in sixth grade sitting in Mr. Schwartz's class. He's writing numbers on the board. The clock strikes 11:30, my time to pick up two kindergartners and take them to their bus to go home. When I get up to leave, I feel ill. Mr. Schwartz sends me to the nurse's office. There's terrible pressure on my head. I start vomiting.

Mom picks me up. She thinks I have the flu and puts me to bed. Then she picks up my sister, Gretch, and my brother, Jim. When she gets back, she asks me, "Do you want something to drink?"

The First Big Boom

*I'm thinking, grape juice, but it comes out garbled,
"Iuyuuhgppp."*

*I can't talk. Mom's eyes grow wide and I get scared. My
voice seems foreign. Grape juice, grape juice, I think,
yelling it now. But it's not me. It's a stranger's mouth
yelling a garbled message, pounding the pillow.*

*Then I'm in an ambulance on my way to the hospital. My
head's going to explode.*

*The doctors are talking to me, but I'm speaking a foreign
language. They say it might be encephalitis. I don't know
what they mean. I'm scared. I want my voice back. They
want me to say the alphabet. I can't. There's pressure on
my back. Feels like a needle pricking me. I'm on my side.
Can't move. Stop. Hurts. There's liquid on my bed. I sit
up.*

"ABCDEFG." Then the doctors disappear.

*I'm back in my own room. Lavender walls. "Grape juice,"
I say. Now it's my mouth saying the words. Faces fade in
and out. Walls disappear. Darkness again.*

Little did I know I would have these same feelings of pain and
confusion 13 years later.

TWO WEEKS LATER—STILL IN A COMA

DENNY

Becki is still in the intensive care unit. Although others have been pretty grave about her ever regaining consciousness, I won't listen. Becki will come out of it. Now I'm surer than ever. She's made it through the grand mal seizures, and all the testing they had to do when we got here. How could I believe otherwise when she also made it through brain surgery and fluid buildup in her lungs?

The doctors called the fluid buildup *Da Nang lung* (a.k.a., shock lung) because it was common with servicemen in Vietnam who had head injuries. She's responding well to the new high pressure respiratory therapy technology, even though the respiratory doctor shocked us by saying he initially questioned if her chance for recovery warranted trying the therapy. How could he even question not trying to save my wife's life!

Yet, what made me most determined was a discussion I had with Becki's father. He approached me in the waiting room and offered his support. He also warned me to be prepared for the worst.

"Becki may never come out of the coma, and if she does, she may be a vegetable. You're still young and have a child now; you won't be able to take care of her and the baby. We may have to think about a place for Becki where they can take care of her needs."

For a moment, I didn't know how to respond to that. I hadn't even considered that as an option, and part of me was a bit angry that he would even suggest such a thing, like he was giving up. I held my tongue, though, when I saw the sadness in his eyes. Faced with the possible loss of his daughter, he was reaching out to me, trying to be helpful. Part of him had come to terms with the reality that Becki might not make it. But I wasn't going to even think about that yet.

"No," I told him and shook my head. "I'll take care of Bec. And I am perfectly confident that Becki will get through this and prove everyone wrong. She has already shown herself to be a fighter, and quite stubborn at that. No one thought she would make it this far, but she has. So, who is to say she won't do it again and come out of the coma? Not me! "

GRETCH

Becki is still in a coma. During this whole time, Mom makes sure Becki looks nice, tending to her nails and face while Dad makes promises of buying her shoes (her favorite obsession), if she'll just wake up. We all talk to her, especially about Aimee, hoping the reminder of her three-month-old daughter will rouse her to consciousness.

On Valentine's Day, Denny brings her a rose, and puts it close to her nose so she can smell it.

Nothing.

Relatives come in every day to help out and wait, hoping for some sign from Becki—some sign that she will come back.

Finally, after weeks of silence, Becki gives us a sign. She moves her fingers ever so slightly. Then she opens her eyes. She has suffered a brain-debilitating stroke and seizures, and fluid build-up in her lungs; she has no muscle control and no signs of independent existence, yet she is awake.

She has come back to us.

A few days later they discharge Becki from the ICU and move her to a general floor.

DENNY

Finally! Becki is out of the ICU and down on a general floor! It's been a long two weeks sitting here in the ICU visitor area and taking turns going in to see her.

It's also been interesting visiting with the family members of other patients in the ICU. We have seen many come and go, some with positive outcomes and others without. We were told that another young lady, about the same age as Becki, came in with a similar AVM hemorrhage the same day Becki did, but did not make it. Hearing things like that makes a lasting impact on us as to how fortunate we are and how grateful we should be to still have Becki. And it provides us a sincere and understanding sense of empathy for the families who had less fortunate outcomes.

Many of the patients in the ICU are coronary bypass patients of the famed heart surgeon, Dudley Johnson, and his colleagues. We observed Dr. Johnson walk in and out of the ICU many times the last month, and it is humbling to witness such breakthrough medical advancements. We learned how a newer more aggressive approach to post-surgery care was such an important part of Dr. Johnson's success. The families we got to know come from all over the U.S. and even some from overseas. The families also took a sincere interest in Becki's situation and were very encouraging and supportive to us.

The First Big Boom

ONE MONTH LATER—BACK WITH THE LIVING, BARELY

BECKI

I feel so weak, like my arms and legs are held down with weights. I can move my fingers, but they feel heavy too. The last thing I remember is being in bed in our apartment. This looks like a hospital. What happened, I wonder. I remember a dream about a baby. It is an awful dream where the baby died. There's a picture of a baby on the table next to me. There are no other pictures there. I don't want to see the baby's photo, but I'm drawn to it. Is it the baby in my dream? The dead baby? I try to get up and push the picture away, but I'm too damned weak. I've lost some of the vision in my right eye. How did that happen? Was I in an accident? I feel so helpless. I have so many questions, but no strength to ask them.

A tall man comes in and sits next to me. He looks familiar, but I can't place him. I can tell he knows me, though, because he kisses me on the forehead and rests his hand on my arm. Maybe we dated or grew up together. I'm not sure, but his eyes are so kind and his smile so warm, I immediately feel at ease with him. And if he knows me, maybe he knows the baby in the picture too.

I grasp for words, but they won't come. I know what I want to ask; I can even see the words I need, but my brain isn't working right. It's like a cruel game of hide and seek and I'm the frustrated loser. A word appears, I reach for it, and then just as quickly, it disappears. If I could only catch them, I could speak them, but I will soon learn that that's not how this game is going to be played. I'm trapped without words so all I can think of to do is turn back to the picture. He picks it up and brings it to me. "Do you know who this is?"

I shake my head, No.

"This is Aimee, our baby girl," he tells me.

I don't believe him. "Baby dead," is all I can manage to blurt out.

"No," he explains, "Aimee's not dead. She's alive. She's at home with your mom right now."

It's too much to take in at once. "No," I cry in frustration. He's lying; I know he is. He rests his hand on my cheek for a moment.

"I'll prove it to you." Then he leaves.

When the sky grows dark, the tall man comes back with a small pink blanket. Pictures flash in my head. First, a baby being brought to me. Then loud crying. Me feeding her and rocking her. And without knowing the rest of our past—however short it was —I know that this baby is mine, and she is alive.

He brings her closer and unravels the blanket. I can see the perfect little face and the tiny pink fingers reaching out to be held. Aimee. I can't express it in words, but I am so grateful that he's brought her to me. I struggle to capture two simple words. This time I find them and hope I sound somewhat coherent. "Baby alive."

"Yes, Aimee's alive," he whispers back, and even with my limited vocabulary, I'm almost positive he can understand me, maybe even read my mind.

* * *

The tall man comes in to see me again. I still don't remember who he is, but I enjoy his visits. While he sits with me, a psychologist joins us and asks me all sorts of questions.

"What's your name?"

A few words, such as my name, are getting easier to catch. "Becki."

"What's the day?"

I look for a calendar but can't find one so I shrug my shoulders.

He holds up four fingers. "How many fingers am I holding up?"

I feel like I am back in school. "One, two."

"How many eyes?"

"One, two."

He writes down something in his notebook. I don't know why this guy bothers me, but he does. I hope he'll leave soon. Next, he checks out my eyesight. He shows me a large piece of paper with letters on it and asks me to read them.

"What is this one?" he asks pointing to the "e."

I know it's an "e," but for some reason, I can't make my mouth form the letter. He tries another letter, then another and another. Still no luck. Those letters are perfectly happy just sitting in my brain. They don't want to take the trip down to my lips.

He writes some more notes, probably that I don't know my ABCs anymore, even though I do. I flatten my hand and pretend to write with the other. "Write," I tell him.

"You want my pen?" he asks.

I nod and he gives me his pen and notebook. "Do," I tell him pointing to the letters. Now I'd show him. He points to the letter "e" again. I grasp the pen and write "e."

The doctor's eyes widen. "How about this one?" He points to the letter "r."

I draw a perfect "r." Just to prove a point, I do three more lines for him. Satisfied, I give him his notebook and pen back and smile contentedly. I am still smart, and I just proved it.

He does one final test before he leaves. I have to follow his fingers with my eyes.

"Look to your left." I look left. "Look to your right." I look right. He moves his finger to the far left. "Can you see it now?"

Yes, I nod. Then he moves his finger to the right.

"Can you see it now?"

Yes, I nod. He moves it farther.

"Can you see it now?"

Yes, I nod. He keeps moving it farther to the right until I can no longer see it.

"Can you see it now?"

I can't see it anymore so I shake my head, No.

He tells me I've lost some of the peripheral vision in my right eye and explains what else happened to me. He says that a lot of people suffer from aphasia—difficulty retrieving words and memories—after going through a trauma such as I just had. He explains that the words and memories are basically trapped inside my head, waiting to be pulled out. But there is another glitch. They aren't in order anymore. Instead, they are stuck up there, broken into tiny pieces, and tossed around like a salad. Now my job is to put it all back together again. I will find out that job is easier said than done.

I close my eyes to absorb everything the psychologist has told me. I have to re-learn everything. But at least now I know what I have to do. I will work tirelessly to get everything that broken vessel robbed me of: control of my body, my voice, and, most of all, my life. My memories play an integral part of that plan, and I ask God to give me the strength to find them.

My parents come in to visit me. I am so glad to see them. Finally familiar faces that I can actually place. I want them to take me home, show me my baby. I want out of here.

The First Big Boom

* * *

The tall man later tells me that, while I was still in the ICU, Dad had gone back to Elgin to get fresh clothes and found that their house had been broken into. The thieve(s) took my Grandpa Miller's mantel clock, pocket watch, and silver coin collection he had given Dad, and also took my Grandma Van's rings and silver place settings she had given Mom.

I feel terrible this happened all because of my being in this stinkin' hospital. Those were special things to Mom and Dad. But I guess there is nothing I can do about bad people who take advantage of other people's unfortunate situations. They never did find the thief or theives, but if I could get out of this place, I would find them and give them a piece of my mind! Mom and Dad, though, had a different perspective on the loss of material things after what they have been through this last month.

* * *

I think whoever's in charge should hire an interior decorator to come in and make this place cozy. There's nothing on the walls except a coat of white paint. My new roommate would appreciate some nice pictures of nature scenes on the walls, too. Maybe it would calm her down so she wouldn't swear so much. I call her the queen of cursing. She swears at the staff. She swears at her food. Then she swears at the air if no one's around. The nurses keep the curtain drawn so I don't have to see her flail about, but listening to her is just as scary.

Wendy, one of the nurse's aides, seems to understand my fear. She tells me my roommate is going through alcohol detox and assures me that the lady won't hurt me. But when things get really bad, Wendy takes her out of the room. She must've talked to someone about the situation too, because a couple days later, I have a new roommate. This time, she is a cancer patient.

My new roommate likes to keep to herself, which is fine with me because I don't feel like talking to anyone anyway. It's too embarrassing. This woman intrigues me, though. She seems regal somehow. Maybe it's the green velvet nightgown she wears with the ruffled collar. Or maybe it's the mass of white hair that cascades down her neck, almost like a princess. There are bald patches interspersed in her hair, but I think she is one of the most striking ladies I've ever seen.

When we're alone, I can hear her groaning in pain and, sometimes, crying. But when her family stops by, her whole appearance changes. Her face brightens and she stops groaning. From the moment they enter the room, especially the young man I assume is her son, her demeanor transforms. She focuses on him so intently that I almost feel like an intruder; that I should leave the room.

The young man is a little apprehensive entering the room, but then quickly goes to her bedside for a hug. They talk quietly, sharing some secret, and then she acknowledges the others. And always, before he leaves, he asks, "When are you coming home?" Her lower lip starts to tremble and then tenses up, but her answer is always the same.

"I'd leave with you now if I could."

Then he looks at her as if trying to comprehend the incomprehensible and goes back to hug her with all his might. He's a young man, but disabled with Down syndrome, I think, with the spirit of a child, but the strength of a man. Knowing how much pain she is in, I wonder how she can bear it. But after he leaves, she relaxes again, lingering in the hug and lost in her memories. Soon she is groaning again, but for a little while that hug had brought her some peace.

The First Big Boom

I hate to admit it, but I am a little jealous of her. Her family and her memories bring her comfort. My family tries to be comforting, but I can see pain in their eyes when I try to make sense of the remembrances they share with me.

* * *

The lady is dead. I can tell because the machine she is hooked up to starts humming. That should signal the nurses and doctors to come, but our room is still empty. Why isn't anyone coming in? I try to speak, but my throat is too tight. I can hardly breathe. Maybe if I could yell, someone would come in and help her. But no one comes, and I can't seem to summon anyone. So, I lie here paralyzed in fear and sadness for what seems like an eternity. Finally, the nurses and doctors come. They pull the curtain, and I can only see shadows hovering over her. One nurse comes to my side.

"Are you okay?" she asks, concern in her eyes.

"Lady died," I say, beginning to cry.

"Yes, she died," the nurse explains. "How would you like to go out for a while?"

"Yes," I nod. I want to get out of here. When I return, the lady is gone.

Later, still shaken, I lie in bed staring at the empty spot where the lady used to be. The tall man comes and sits next to me. He must know the lady is gone too because he doesn't ask. I need to talk about it, though. "She died," I tell him. "She died."

"Who?" the tall man asks as if he doesn't know.

"My lady."

"The one next to you?"

I nod and cry some more. I don't like this place. I don't want to be around death when I am struggling to live.

Hernzebekana! Her Language of Love

* * *

"Home?" I ask my parents at their next visit.

"In a little while," they reassure me. "The doctors aren't ready to let Denny take you home yet."

"Denny," I repeat in my mind, trying to make his name stick in my head. For some reason, I can't say his name. I know he's my husband, but the name "Denny" keeps slipping from my mind. Other pieces of the picture stick with me though, like the crib in the living room, our bedroom, and him grabbing his coffee as he heads out the door for school.

But that can't be all there is. He tells me we've been married for two years, so where are all the missing pieces? And when will I be able to say my own husband's name? I hope it will be before I have to go home with him. My whole body fills with dread at that thought. I have to go home with him as his wife. His wife, for God's sake, and I can't even remember the tall man's name. See, I forgot it again. Now how is this going to work?

***

The next time Mom comes to visit me I ask her for my purse. I have this feeling there is something in there that I need. Mom looks at me curiously, wondering what the heck I have this sudden need for. I fiddle around inside each purse compartment; then suddenly come upon the craving I was having—my Virginia Slims menthols! Mom communicates her dismay by grabbing them and placing them out of my reach. In a familiar voice that brought me back to my childhood, she says, "You don't need those anymore!" I can see that look in the eyes of my Scotch-Irish, registered nurse mother—and I realize I'm not going to win this discussion. Little did I know that would be the last time I ever touched a cigarette.

The First Big Boom

* * *

There should be a law against good-looking nurses in the hospital. Especially when you yourself are bald (Dad had shaved my whole head so I wouldn't look so lopsided.), feeling ugly, and not having had a decent bath in a month. (Sponge baths don't count.) Which brings me to the subject of Nurse Lila.

You wouldn't think a nurse's uniform would be sexy, but believe me, on her, it is. Her white starched uniforms are always perfect, her hair set in a flawless bob that plays up her high cheekbones and porcelain skin. She smells like expensive perfume, and she thinks my husband is the most interesting thing she's ever laid eyes on. Just perfect.

I knew she was trouble the first time she came in with the rest of her class (did I mention she's a nurse in training?). Well, anyway, while everyone is talking to me, I see her noticing my husband. She spends the whole session studying my husband when she should be studying me.

The next few times she comes in, she makes sure to spend a few minutes engaging the tall man in idle chit-chat and flashing him that great big smile of hers. I could be having a seizure on the bed and she wouldn't notice. One time, she comes in the room and asks the tall man if I want juice. She sits down next to him, looks him straight in the eye, flashes him one of those big smiles, and asks, "Does she want any juice?"

Hello! I want to shout at her, I may have brain damage, but that doesn't make me invisible. Talk to me, (and I know you have the hots for my husband). I am so angry, I wave my arms at her and say more firmly than I had said anything since I woke up, "Here."

When she comes over, I glare at her. "Talk...to...me." She doesn't say too much after that, but does bring me a big glass of grape juice.

After everyone leaves, I stew in my anger for a bit. I haven't felt like this in a long time. And I discover I am more than angry, I am jealous. That woman was flirting with my husband and I don't like it, not one bit. The tall man is mine, even if our times together are still foggy, he is mine.

DENNY

She hasn't said my name yet. She's called me Mike and Jake, Steve and Tim—apparently some of her old boyfriends! Once she got close and called me Lenny. I don't make a big deal of it because I know she's trying. If not, she has a new boyfriend every time I visit.

Today, I ask Becki if I can join her in her bed. It is about 4 p.m., and she is lying in bed with her feet propped up. I think she is trying to put the bed down, so I asked if I could lie next to her. She hesitates for a moment and then nods. We stay like this for most of the evening, just listening to each other breathe.

BECKI

The tall man asked if he could lie next to me tonight. I tell him to turn the light out first, in case we fall asleep. He tries telling me it isn't bedtime, but that's hard to believe. It seems like bedtime. It's dark outside and I'm tired, so it must be. He keeps trying to explain the time, but he finally gives up and just hops into the bed. Then he helps me put my bed back down. (I have such a hard time maneuvering the controls with my hands; they're still pretty weak.) I am a little apprehensive when he scoots in next to me, but once he is beside me, it just seems right. Just the two of us matching breaths in the quietness of the night.

Maybe lying next to each other has helped jog my brain. The name "Denny" is now becoming more familiar to me. I can now think his name in my mind, but I still can't say it out loud. I just can't slide those letters D-E-N-N-Y out of my mouth into a word yet. I guess we're making progress. I will just need to figure out how to get my brain to send the letters down to my mouth in one piece.

BECKI

All I want is chicken, but no one will get it for me. No one's being mean to me; they just can't understand what I'm saying. I can see a scrumptious fried chicken in my head, on a nice plate of wild rice, and it makes my mouth water. Maybe that's the problem; my mouth is watering and I need to swallow. I swallow and try again.

"Baa gaa." No, that's not right. I try again.

"Aaah gaa." Dad is staring at me trying to decipher the real meaning of those words.

Mom decides to start guessing. "You want sherbet?" (I've lived on sherbet for the past few weeks, mostly orange.)

I grimace and shake my head, No. Now everyone follows suit and starts guessing.

"A sandwich?" asks Dad.

"Ice cream?" asks Denny.

"Something to drink?" asks Mom.

No, no, no! I grab the pad of paper and pen at the side of my bed and start writing the word *chicken*, but it comes out looking like continual ovals. I give up on the letters and start drawing the chicken. It's a very rough version of a drumstick with a balloon thigh leading into a squared bone at the bottom. Dad studies the picture like it's a college exam. He furrows his brows and tries to find the right answer.

"Looks like a mug of soup." Then he checks with me to see if he got it right.

I sigh and shake my head again. I'll probably starve before they figure this one out.

"That's not soup," my mom corrects him, "That's a hamburger with a pickle on the side."

I roll my eyes. Wrong again. Denny takes the piece of paper and gives it a try.

"Is it steak?"

I groan. How could they think it was anything but a chicken? It's not the best depiction of a chicken leg but it's also not modern art, for heaven's sake! I fold my arms and flap them like a bird and shout, "*Bawck, bawck!*" Then everyone's roaring.

"You want chicken!" my dad laughs.

"She's always been resourceful," says Mom proudly, writing chicken on my dinner order for the nurse. I lie back and smile. I won't starve after all.

The First Big Boom

TWO MONTHS LATER—MAKING PROGRESS

DENNY

I ask Becki if she wants to look through our photo album. When she nods, I bring the book closer and start flipping through the pages, explaining all the pictures—where we were and what we were doing. And I don't leave out any details, trying to paint the whole picture for her, right down to our conversations, hoping it will trigger something and make her see me like she used to.

Every time I point to a new picture, it's as if we've gone back in time, reliving that very moment. I'm no longer her husband but her boyfriend, and we're on a date, getting reacquainted with each other, except this time I know how the story ends.

"That me?" Becki asks pointing to the girl in the purple top and matching pants. I nod.

"Yep, that picture was taken at my fraternity party the night we started dating." I look for signs of recognition on her face, but instead she looks at me like a child at storytime waiting for the next page to be read.

"You had already gone on dates with two of my fraternity brothers. That night it was my turn to try and impress you. First there was Frank, but I don't think you liked him that much. Then there was Tom. He was the one I had to worry about because I knew you thought he was a nice guy."

Becki laughs at this idea.

Encouraged, I continue. "That night was movie night at the fraternity house, and we were showing a Western movie. We had pizza and popcorn and a half-barrel of beer on tap. You, of course, wanted something classier than beer. You wanted a whiskey sour. So, to really impress you, I had one of the guys

41

show me how to make one. That was the most meticulously perfect drink I ever made. It had to be because you needed to be more impressed with me than with Frank or Tom."

"Whiskey sour is good." She nods and runs her fingers over the picture. Now it's my turn to laugh.

"Yeah, you used to joke that that drink sealed the deal. Then I'd kid you back and say it was those tan legs and that miniskirt you wore so often in Doc Suttle's English class that did it for me."

There's a little glimmer in Becki's eye as she turns the page over and points to the next picture.

"Tell more." Becki smiles at me, eager to hear more of her story.

"All three of us were in the same English class with you, and Tom was on the football team with me. The only reason I can think of that you picked me was that I made the best whisky sour that night."

BECKI

He's doing it again! Denny takes me in a wheelchair down to the hospital chapel. He thinks it will be good for me, and he even says a prayer for us while we are there. I know this is probably a good idea, but right now I think I am mad at God for what has happened to me and I'm not sure I want to be here. But I don't have a choice since I am the one in the wheelchair and Denny is the one operating it.

I know I shouldn't be mad at God, but maybe I can blame it on my brain not functioning properly. One thing I do remember from all my years in church is that God can handle it—my being mad at him that is. And I do know that he cares about me and will take care of me. I say a little prayer to myself that hopefully my attitude will change when I get better.

Denny tells me about the schedule he and Mom have set up while he still goes to school and they both take care of Aimee. Mom comes up and helps me with breakfast early in the morning. If Denny has to head to school before Mom gets home, he drops Aimee off with some friends in our building until Mom gets home.

When Denny comes home late afternoon, Mom comes up to see me and helps with my supper while he feeds and plays with Aimee. When Mom goes back to the apartment, Denny comes up to the hospital to see me for the evening. Sometimes he gets away around noon or early afternoon and comes to see me then. Sometimes, when Denny can't get home, Mom drops Aimee off with our friends in the building. It sounds like they really have it down to a science—kinda like handing off a baton in a relay race. Of course, with Denny being a scientist and having run track in high school and college, I guess that makes sense.

GRETCH

Becki's not in her room! What happened? It takes only a few minutes of panic to discover she was given permission to go home and eat dinner with Denny, Mom, and Dad. Hooray! Mom must have wanted to surprise us because I thought she knew that Jim and I, and Jim and Becky, were coming up from Illinois to visit Becki.

As we enter their apartment, we all rush to get our hands on Becki. She accepts our hugs graciously, and tries to hug back, but she is still very weak. Her skin is pale and her body has lost its softness. Her features are now more angular and sharper from all the weight she has lost. But her eyes are the same. They sparkle with that old fire that Becki had before all this happened.

Then I know she is on her way back.

BECKI

Getting back to our apartment is like walking through a maze. *Watch out for the steps, walk around the table, look out for the lamp,* etc.

But the gold shag carpeting is the worst. It's like walking through a swamp trying not to get stuck. If I don't lift my feet high enough, I will trip and sink right into the floor. So, I hold onto Denny and concentrate on the movements of my legs. Bring my knee up to my belly, bring it back down. Do the same with my other foot. I repeat these directions in my head until I am sitting on the couch.

Even though I'm exhausted sitting here, I'm happier than I've been in weeks. I am home. I am no longer confined to the bleached white walls of the hospital and the buzzing and beeping of machines. I'm surrounded by colors and softness and the clanking of dishes as my family lovingly prepares my first meal at home.

When the meal is on the table, Denny offers his arm and we go to sit down together. Although the mood is light, and everyone is acting like things are back to normal, I can read their eyes. This is a test. Am I well enough to come home for good? I wonder the same thing, and hope I pass.

The First Big Boom

At first, I just watch my family go through the process of filling their plates. I wonder what I should choose and how much I should put on my plate. I watch Denny carefully. Denny puts his napkin on his lap; I copy him. Denny takes a slice of meatloaf, so I do the same. He picks up a medium-sized baked potato and sets it on his plate. I also choose a potato and place it on my plate. Then I panic. *How do I eat this thing?*

DENNY

I know Becki is watching me trying to figure out how to eat like everyone else. Then I realize that I am now not only Becki's husband, but her teacher also. I slow down and wait for her to copy me. I can tell she's not sure about the potato so I pick up my knife and cut it in half lengthwise. Becki picks up her knife and does the same. I glance at her so she doesn't know I'm watching and then make smaller cuts along the body of the potato.

BECKI

So that's how it works! Steam pours out of Denny's potato and that's when it hits me. I eat the white stuff inside. I cut open my potato and smell the aroma. I haven't enjoyed these smells—smells from food that's just been cooked in the kitchen—since I left our apartment that fateful morning two months ago.

Denny picks up his knife and takes a small slice of butter and drops it on the inside of his potato. Next, he puts a few spoonfuls of green beans on his plate and begins eating. There is a small bowl next to our plates. Denny hasn't put anything in it and I wonder what it's for.

I scan the table and focus on the plate of lime-green Jell-O. I remember the Jell-O as one of my favorite dishes that Mom always made for me on special occasions. Pear halves form a circle around the Jell-O. And I know a treasure of cream cheese balls are hidden behind those pears. My mouth starts to water as I remember how tart the fruit tasted but the cream cheese was rich.

I wanted to have some of that, but Denny didn't take any! Now how was I supposed to politely get it? I keep my head forward so he won't know I'm watching him, but I study him from the corner of my eye and wait.

DENNY

Oh, yeah, Becki always takes a scoop of Jell-O first. I know she won't eat anything until she gets that Jell-O so I forget about my green beans for the moment and scoop out a piece and drop it into my bowl.

BECKI

Finally! I grab the spoon after Denny's done and take a big portion of the jiggly, heavenly, Jell-o salad. Now everything is in its place, and I can start eating too.

Among the whir of conversation, I tune in and out, trying to concentrate on what I'm doing. It feels like I'm at a tennis match watching words fly past me too fast to comprehend. They talk about Aimee and how big she's getting, Gretch's teaching job, Denny's thesis on hydrogeology, and so on.

Dad says to me, "Bec, we're having raspberry or orange sherbet for dessert. Which one do you want?"

I look at him in disbelief, hoping we won't be having that gosh-awful sherbet AGAIN. Then Dad winks at me, and I know it's going to be something better. Sure enough, Mom walks in with a homemade apple pie, one of my favorites. And everything seems normal as hell, whatever that is.

After dinner, Denny takes me back to the hospital. He puts his arms around me and we share a lingering kiss. "Soon, Bec," he whispers before he leaves. I nod at him. I finally feel like I have a future, and not a bad one at that.

As I lie in the darkness with only the shuffling of nurses walking in and out to keep me company, I have time to reevaluate the night. I know I have more work to do before I can be discharged. Physically and mentally I'm still not prepared to leave the security of my hospital room. But I'm determined to get stronger.

First thing the next morning, I ask for more physical therapy. I set my goal. I'll be home by Easter. The physical therapist works with me an hour and a half in the morning and then again in the afternoon. We work on getting the muscle tone back in my right leg. She makes me wrap two-pound weights on both my ankles. Then she asks me to get on all four limbs like a dog.

"Okay Becki, I want you to lift your left arm." Even though it looks ridiculous, I follow her instructions.

"Now, Becki, lift your right leg up."

I pause for a second and picture this position in my head and realize I'm going to fall on my ass! I look at my therapist with an expression that says, *You've got to be kidding*. She waits. She's not kidding at all. She really wants me to do this, which means I have to figure out how to make it work. Gathering all the strength I can muster; I lift up my right leg and that's when the inevitable happens. I fall on my ass.

As I'm lying on my back staring at the ceiling tiles, she says, "Becki, that was wonderful! Let's try it again."

I really hate this woman.

DENNY

Becki has been doing so well in her recovery, and then all of a sudden, she seems to have a setback. She is more confused and lethargic about things and isn't interested in eating. The doctors are perplexed. They tell us it can be a roller coaster ride but still don't know what is going on right now. Her mom and I try to figure out what might be going on, then we remember that the doctors recently stopped one of her medications, the Decadron, which is a steroid that is used to address inflammation in the brain.

We tell the doctors that this is the only thing we can think of that has changed recently, so they decide to put her back on the Decadron. Boy! Within a day she starts bouncing back better than ever! This teaches us how important the observations of loved ones can be in helping with the medical treatment of patients.

The First Big Boom

APRIL 12, 1976—FINALLY GOING HOME

BECKI

Denny's taking me home today. Midmorning, Denny helps me put my clothes on and get ready to leave. He picks up my suitcase while a nurse brings a wheelchair for me. I feel like a queen as I'm pushed to all the different departments to say goodbye.

At each stop, nurses and doctors greet me with hugs and a few tears.

"Don't forget us," they tell me.

I nod and thank each person, knowing I will never be able to forget them: the night nurse who made sure I wasn't frightened by the hallucinogenic ranting coming from the patient next to me; Dr. Uttech and Dr. Becker, who explained my situation to me and never condescended, and everyone else who made sure I was comfortable.

They were there when I came out of the darkness and they were there to rehabilitate me, befriend me, and help me become a part of the world again. It's almost surreal leaving these people on whom I have come to depend for more than two months now. And as much as I want to leave the sterile atmosphere of the hospital, I almost hope someone will throw me a lifeline, pull me back inside, and tell me my room is still there if I need it.

Then the hospital doors open and a cool breeze filled with the soft, musky smell of spring flowers envelopes me. It seems as if everything is fresh and new. Denny leans forward and whispers, "You ready for this?"

I pat his hand and nod. I am now.

When we get to the apartment, Mom is waiting with Aimee. First thing I want to do is hold my baby and tell her I love her, but she wants no part of that. It's worse than her not even acknowledging me; she doesn't want me.

I'm her mother and she wants nothing to do with me. I can't blame her, though. I have become a stranger to her. While I was gone, my mother filled in for me and developed a strong bond with Aimee, that mother-daughter bond that was rightfully mine. Still, I can't expect Aimee to jump right back into my arms. I'll have to earn that honor back. Feeling defeated, I put my hands down and give my mom a kiss instead. Aimee begins to cry, and I have to swallow hard not to join her.

"It'll just take time," Mom reassures me.

I muster a smile. "I know," I tell her. "That's something I still have. Time."

* * *

The next day, Mom begins her own method of physical therapy with me. That evil physical therapist from the hospital could've taken lessons from MY mom! Mom not only continues the therapies I was subjected to at the hospital, she breathes life into them, making it a matter of survival. (I have a sneaking suspicion that Mom has become the devil incarnate while I was gone. Sometimes, when she is eating, I swear I see a red tail swishing behind her seat, but that is probably my imagination, right?)

Mom's therapeutic philosophy is simple: get off your butt and do it yourself. I can hardly argue with her, so I get up. That first morning together, Mom looks at me from across the kitchen counter.

"Do you want something for breakfast?"

"Yes," I reply and wait for Mom to find something. Mom stares back at me.

"What would you like?"

The First Big Boom

I think for a moment. Eggs seem the logical choice because it would be the easiest to say, but after I say it, everything is downhill. I soon find out that that isn't the end of it. Mom is going to make me prepare it.

"Well," says Mom. "You know where the eggs are."

You've got to be kidding, I think. I have no idea where they are. They could still be in the chicken for all I know. And, excuse me, but I do have brain damage. Can't I get a little break because of it? Isn't a mother supposed to help you?

Mom looks away, and I know that's my answer. I'm on my own, and she's waiting for me to make the next move.

Stay calm, I tell myself. If you were an egg, where would you be? Maybe the cabinets? I check each one, still no egg. Next, I search the counters, the bread drawer, and lastly, the refrigerator. Thank God, there they are. I feel like I've found a lost treasure as I proudly take it to Mom for inspection.

"Egg," I tell her.

Mom nods. "Is it done?"

Is it done? Crap, now I have to make it too? I search for a bowl. It's in the cabinet. I make a mental note of that and place it on the counter. Would she help me now? I glance her way and notice that she's trying to keep occupied wiping the table. Without taking her eyes off the table, she asks, "What will you cook it in?"

I look around. A pan. I need a pan. I go on another search and find it in the drawer next to the sink. Then I'm stuck. I stand there looking at the egg, the bowl, and the pan. From one to the other and back again, not knowing where to begin.

Finally, Mom asks, "Do you want some help?"

Relieved that she's finally stepping in, I exhale and say, "Yes."

"Becki, you just have to ask." Mom puts her arm around my shoulders and gives me a reassuring squeeze. "Then I'll help." She smiles at me but then it's back to therapy. "Now, how do you want it?"

Mom offers a suggestion, testing me. "Scrambled? Fried?"

I shrug my shoulders. It doesn't matter. I just want to make whatever is the easiest. I choose fried. Then I'm guided through every painstaking step, every movement, every decision. Which hand to use. How to crack the egg. Flip it. And finally, place it on my plate. Mom also helps me make some toast and spreads the butter on it.

"Do you want some fruit?"

I shake my head, No. Much easier to just have toast and an egg. I am finally getting smart at this game. It will be much easier to prepare less, and then no one will have to see me fumble through the steps, especially me.

After all the hard work of actually making the meal, I find out my stomach has trouble digesting this food that has been foreign to my body for so long.

I throw up everything.

Eating homemade food is something I'll have to get used to. Next time, I'll have oatmeal, like Aimee. Exhausted, I sit down on the couch and rest.

CHAPTER 4

THE JOURNEY BACK

BECKI

After a couple weeks being back at our small apartment, Denny and my folks think it might be best for Aimee and me to go back to my parents' home in Elgin just until I can take care of myself and Aimee again. Mom has been in our small apartment in Milwaukee for almost three months now and I think she is homesick. Plus with both Mom and Dad there and a bigger home I am familiar with, it is just a better setting to help my recovery.

While I'm with my parents, Denny will be at the university finishing up his last semester of classes and working on his master's thesis. He will come to visit on weekends.

It's weird not having a place of our own anymore, almost as if the last few years have been erased. But looking at Aimee, I know that's not true. She's proof that I AM a mother and a wife, and that I will fill those roles again. I have to. This clueless person who's taken over my body must leave. I have a child to take care of.

MAY 1976—A SPRING STROLL

VELDA (A.K.A. MOM)

It's such a beautiful spring morning, flowers are starting to rise from their winter slumber and peek out of the earth. Outside our kitchen window, I can see two robins busily pulling strands of grass to place in some hidden nest.

Becki has finished dressing and Aimee has eaten nearly all that is left of her rice cereal and mashed peaches. I try the airplane trick to encourage her to finish her food—*whoosh, whoosh*—but she'll have none of it. She's ready for playtime.

Becki seems a bit frustrated with Aimee and looks at her sternly and says, "Eat the bowling." Hmm! It might not be the correct word, but she seems to get the point across and Aimee starts eating the rest of her food. I guess we will need to get used to some of Becki's new vocabulary, but she is starting to understand her role as a mother.

Becki kisses Aimee's head and turns to me.

"Ready?" she asks.

"Ready," I tell her and then I clean Aimee up.

We start the slow trek outside with Aimee in tow. Becki takes slow, deliberate steps behind me while I set Aimee in her buggy and push her outside. I make sure I hold the door open once I'm out so Becki can focus on the three steps that lead out of our front door onto Ryerson Avenue.

The morning is more luxurious than I thought it would be. The air is warm with the promise of summer and I begin to point out all the wonderful colors that are sprouting from the small patches of landscaped yards. I guess I'm chattering more than I should because Becki puts her hand on my arm.

"No," she tells me. "No talk."

I'm puzzled as she gathers her thoughts to explain why. "I walk."

Then I understand. Becki needs to concentrate on walking and nothing else. Silently, I slow down my stride to match Becki's. She struggles to walk less abruptly, more fluidly. The sidewalk is much different than the few steps she must take in our home, and her legs are as unsteady as a colt's just learning to keep itself up. She puts one foot forward and shifts her weight to that leg. Then she repeats the process with her other foot. Finally, she's made it a few yards. She looks up at me triumphantly and turns around.

My mind drifts back to the time Becki was in sixth grade, lying sick in a hospital bed, and couldn't form the words she wanted to say to me.

She wanted grape juice, I knew, but instead she said, "Giffjaa."

I knew something was terribly wrong then, but the doctors couldn't tell us what it was. Some sort of viral infection like encephalitis they thought, but no answer was concrete.

Then, when she was finally released from the hospital because she could speak and say her alphabet again, she looked at me with that same triumphant smile as she did this time.

My heart is breaking for her. I want to hold her in my arms and reassure her that it will all be okay. But she needs to do this on her own. I smile back at her when what I really want to do is cry.

THE DINNER ADVENTURE

BECKI

After another long day of therapy with Mom, playing the Simon electronic board game (which challenges my visual skills, memory, and hand movement), walking, and then practicing my conversational skills, I am ready for a relaxing dinner.

But I should've known nothing would ever be relaxing for me again. My therapy that day culminates in my helping Mom prepare the meal. Although Mom does most of the preparation, I help with the smaller jobs like cleaning the potatoes, scrubbing them, and putting them in a pan so they can go in the oven.

Mom never seems to run out of things for me to do—get the plates and utensils out, wipe the table, and rip the lettuce apart—all in the name of improving my eye-hand coordination.

I get a little reprieve because I also have to take care of Aimee. I can tell Mom is doing less and less for Aimee so that I will do more. This scares me more than anything. I enjoy holding my child, but I don't feel ready to care for all her needs yet. So, I handle her like a China doll, always aware of her fragility and mine, not wanting to break either of us.

"Dinner's ready," Mom says as she places everything on the kitchen counter. "And the potatoes look great," she says triumphantly. "You did a good job, Bec."

I nod and rock Aimee. I am tired, so tired, but I smile because it is Friday and Denny is coming for the weekend.

The Journey Back

DENNY

Bec looks so tired. I hate to see her so drained. I know it'll take time for her to regain her strength, but I wish I could be the one to stay with her and Aimee. I miss them so much during the week, but I know I have to finish school. I don't know what financial challenges Becki's condition will bring, so finishing school and getting a job are important for us to have a future and stay out of debt. So, every Monday, I kiss my wife and child goodbye, put my emotions aside and focus on the job: finish school and get my family back.

"Hi, Babe," I say and kiss Bec. She smiles up at me, but still doesn't say my name.

BECKI

He's home!

Just seeing his face erases all the anxiety of the day. I watch him take Aimee into his arms, cherishing the smell of her baby skin and the way she snuggles into his neck.

I thought Denny had wanted to get away from me, his invalid wife. After all, what good was I to him? What good was I to anybody anymore? But the gentle kiss he gives me and the way he holds Aimee tells me that I might be wrong. Maybe being away from us all week is as hard on him as it is on me.

Soon, Dad's home and we're all sitting at the table ready for a nice home-cooked meal. Mom passes each of us a plate already filled with food. I'm relieved that she does this because I won't have to make as many choices during the meal. All of us have a portion of meat, a potato, and a stalk of broccoli on our plates. The only item I'll have to deal with is the salad.

Mom sets a big bowl of lettuce on the table for us to pass around. Then she grabs two glass containers, one filled with a red liquid and one with creamy yellow stuff. I study each one and try to remember where they're supposed to go. After we pray, we begin eating. No one is starting with the salad or the potato, so I have no one to copy at the moment. My salad bowl remains empty as I check to see what everyone is doing. Denny's cutting up his meat; Dad's chewing on a piece of broccoli; Mom's taking a sip of wine, and Aimee, well, she's mushing the broccoli between her fingers and then shoving it in her face. Sometimes I wish I could do that!

Since I really want some salad, I ask Denny to pass the salad bowl. He hands it to me and I fill my bowl with the lettuce. Next is the tricky part. Which container should I use? I figure I have a fifty-fifty chance of getting it right, so I grab the container with the creamy yellow stuff. It looks pretty appetizing to me as I spread a generous amount over my lettuce.

Denny looks at my bowl, a little revolted, I think, and says, "Bec, hon, what we usually do is put the butter on the potato and the dressing on the salad."

He offers me the red liquid instead. I shake my head and push his hand away.

"No," I tell him. I'm sick and tired of all this stuff, trying to remember what goes where, trying to pull things out of my brain to say, trying to be what I used to be. I may have hated staying in the hospital, but at least it was easier there. This was just plain humiliating, and I was tired of it all.

"Like it that way," I tell him defiantly and eat the whole buttery thing.

The Journey Back

SUMMER 1976—THE CHECKUP

BECKI

This morning, my task is to put on makeup for our trip to Milwaukee to meet Dr. Uttech. It will be the first time I've seen the doctor since I left the hospital two months ago. After applying the lipstick for the third time, I finally have it right. Just enough on my lips, and no excess bleeding on the surrounding skin. My blush and eye liner are now muted and soft, leaving the reflection in the mirror looking more elegant and less garish than it has in past attempts.

I stand for a moment and admire my work. Since leaving the hospital, I have struggled to take care of myself: put my bra on without falling, pull my underwear up over my hips so the front is in the front and the back is in the back, pick an outfit for the day, and make meals that don't just depend on a can opener, spoon, and bowl.

Old dreams of continuing my education are now replaced by dreams of making it through the day without having to ask my mom for help, and now I am finally succeeding. I do it all by myself—no one peering over my shoulder, waiting to guide my hands in the right direction.

Looking over the whole ensemble, I have to admit, I really pulled it off today. The navy-blue bandana adorning my head and covering the tufts of brown hair growing underneath, looks stylish and neat. The image in the mirror smiles back at me. This woman looks more like the woman I remember—the one I yearn to become again. This woman is smart, pretty, and confident, just like the college kid at Valparaiso University. But when I look closer—at her dark eyes and the pale cheeks hidden behind blush and drawn close to the bone from months in a bed—I realize it's only a facade.

I touch the face and wonder how long it will be before I feel whole again. But the image doesn't answer me. The woman staring back at me now is no longer smiling, her expression less confident and more like that of a scared little girl.

VELDA

On the way to Milwaukee, Aimee starts screaming. I look into the rearview mirror and watch Becki's reaction. There is none. She continues to stare out the window entranced by the moving landscape. I pull over at a rest stop to calm Aimee down and wonder how long it will be until Becki can take care of herself and her child.

"Stop?" Becki asks.

"Mmm hmm," I nod, and pull the keys out of the ignition. "Aimee needs a little break."

Becki watches me as I unbuckle Aimee and take her outside for some fresh air. She watches us as we walk away, but then closes her eyes and rests her head back on the seat. In a few weeks, Denny will be done with school, get a job, and start to set up their own home somewhere. Then what will happen to Becki and Aimee? But I have to get rid of these thoughts. Besides, it's not my place to say anything. They'll just have to make it work.

Aimee relaxes in my arms so I gently put her back in the car. Both my babies are fast asleep.

The Journey Back

BECKI

Once at the doctor's office, Denny is waiting for us at the entrance. When Aimee sees him, she holds up her arms and is scooped up and covered with kisses. He looks a little tired, probably from all the work he's been doing to finish his thesis in hydrogeology.

Hydrogeology. I can hardly say the word, yet my husband is specializing in it. It makes me wonder what we even have in common anymore. Me—the one who can't even say his name, and him—the one who can write a fifty-page thesis on the groundwater supply within the Mequon, Wisconsin, area.

What does he see when he looks at me now? The pretty woman in the mirror or the scared little girl?

"Well, let's see what the doc has to say," Denny says and holds out his other hand to me. I brush aside all the negative thoughts and focus on what's ahead. Whatever Denny sees doesn't seem to matter right now. All that matters is that we're together, and he's taking care of me.

DENNY

Becki looks good all dressed up. Such a difference from the way she was in the hospital. Looking at her, with color on her cheeks and her hair pushing out from underneath the bandana, I remember the girl I fell in love with, and the night we sat and cuddled into the early morning hours underneath a grand old oak tree at Valpo. The tree had to be at least fifty years old and spread itself out next to the social studies building. A sidewalk drew a dividing

61

line between the tree and the building and allowed students to pass by, some clasping books to their chest and running, some just walking and thinking.

Becki and I had a lot to think about, then. Like lovers in that old song, *Under the Old Oak Tree*, Becki and I would meet to watch the sun and moon trade places. We'd lie back and look up at the leaves dancing above us and make plans for our future, sneaking kisses when we thought no one was looking. It was our junior year and we were getting married before we started our senior year.

After the wedding, our plan was that we'd take turns going back to school for our master's degrees. I'd get mine first and then Becki would go back for her law degree. She wanted to specialize in children's cases while I looked for groundwater.

Then a house—nothing too extravagant, two children, and maybe the dog she wanted. It was the perfect plan.

I can still see the graceful curved branches of the oak tree swaying carelessly against the darkening sky paying no attention to the social studies building with its stiff lines organized in intricate detail just a few yards away from it.

I look through the clinic doors and wish I didn't have to step inside. I'd rather take Becki back to our old oak tree and stare up into the whispering leaves with its carefree dance and our perfect plan laid out in front of us. The song *Colour My World* starts up in my head. I had practiced it for weeks on the piano just so I could play it for Becki when we got serious about each other. I longed for that image of Becki standing before me as I played it for her, dark wisps of hair framing her glistening eyes, beaming at me, our whole future in front of us.

But then reality hits me and I'm pulled back to the present by Becki's gentle touch. She looks at me, confused, her soft fingers wrapped in mine. I have to will myself forward, out of the old perfect plan, through the door, and wait for God to give us HIS new plan.

BECKI

I'm not sure I want to see Dr. Uttech again. Part of me fears that if I walk through those doors, they might send me back to the hospital. What if they think I'm not okay, not normal enough to walk back out?

An image I have long since pushed into my subconscious now appears. It is the elegant lady in the green robe in my hospital room. She is lying in her bed, crying softly, and staring out the window. She's all alone, while outside her window, people are walking by taking no notice. The sun is streaming onto the lady's face, but it's not her face anymore.

It's mine.

My stomach knots up, and I try to shake the image. I have to remind myself that I survived. I can talk, although not well yet, and I can walk. And if I want, I can just as easily walk out. I am determined to make everyone see that I am healed. I am normal. The Bec is back!

Down the hall, Dr. Uttech steps out of his office to see what all the commotion is about. When I see the expression on his face, I know he is impressed. We stare at each other for a moment and then he smiles, waiting for me to walk to him. This is my test. I grab hold of Denny's arm and head towards Dr. Uttech.

When I finally stand in front of him, he shakes my hand and motions for me to join him in the office.

"You look well."

"Thank you."

I don't want him to think less of my recovery by speaking, so I decide to say as little as possible. Hopefully less talk will help me appear more normal.

After a few routine questions, he asks me to walk a straight line for him. Each step is so slow and laborious without Denny's steady hand to catch me if I fall. I feel like a drunk walking a straight line for a police officer—not that I ever experienced that, of course!

Once I make it to the other side of the room, I heave a sigh of relief and sit down.

Satisfied with the exercise, Dr. Uttech examines my eyes.

"Your right eye is still the same," he says, scribbling something down on his clipboard.

His handwriting looks like chicken scratches and I find some satisfaction in knowing that even if I could read, I wouldn't be able to read his notes. I nod in agreement, but say nothing.

"I'd like to see you again in a month, when I also want to take a picture of your brain with a new type of x-ray machine called a CAT scan. I'm very pleased with your progress."

Another nod and the meeting is over. I take Denny's hand and walk back to the reception area where Aimee and Mom are waiting.

Now I know how to compensate for my disability. I promise myself I will work hard and regain everything I can, but any weaknesses will be hidden and stay hidden until I can fix them myself.

I know I'm testing my luck, but I decide to stop at the hospital and say hello to all the people who were so much a part of my life for two months. And since I know Dr. Uttech isn't going to stick me back in the hospital, it is a safe place to visit. But nothing could have prepared me for the reception I receive when we enter the hospital. It is like a family reunion, awkward at first with everyone quiet, followed by hugs and, "You look wonderful!" or "How you've changed!" A steady stream of nurses, doctors, and candy stripers swarm me from all different directions. I didn't expect this. It is as if I am a celebrity.

That's when I realize they had expectations too. From the start they expected me to die that first night. Then, they expected me to sleep the rest of my life away in a coma. It is as if I have my own cheering section rooting for me, glad for every expectation I have thwarted. Now standing here, I see the hope in their eyes and realize how miraculous my recovery must be to them, and it gives me strength.

THE TENNIS GAME

BECKI

My sister, Gretch, and her husband, Jim, come for the weekend. We decide to get out of the house for a while and play tennis.

I'm quite familiar with the tennis courts because every weekend Denny lobs tennis balls at me trying to improve my hand-eye coordination. After getting a couple bruises the first few rounds, I figured out that I need to keep my body angled slightly forward so I can keep the ball within my field of vision. I can't see very far to the right side, so if I stay forward, I won't lose sight of the ball.

This time, I'm ready to hit the courts and show Gretch what I can do, but after a few frustrating swipes, I drop the racket on the sidelines and sit, me and my self-pity, on the bleachers. Denny and Jim continue playing a real tennis match.

Gretch joins me. She's staring at her feet, and I can tell there's something she wants to say, but she's not sure how to approach it. I wait in dread wondering what's going to come out of her mouth. Maybe a reprimand for playing so lousy or just for quitting. Whatever it is, I don't want to hear it. Finally, she lifts her head and speaks, but she's not looking at me. She remains expressionless, talking to the space in front of her, not me.

"You can say 'Denny' correctly if you try."

Then her concentration turns to the little yellow ball flying across the net. Her eyes follow, never leaving the rhythm of the ball as it goes back and forth from one side to the other. I can feel a knot tightening in my stomach.

"Can't," I tell her, tight-lipped, hoping that would be the end of it.

But Gretch doesn't give up easily, and I know she won't let this go. She can be quite stubborn. And the more she presses the issue, the more I object. She hasn't seen the times before when I did try to say his name, but it comes out as a stranger's or worse yet, all scrambled up making me sound like a child, not the full-grown woman I am.

At first Denny was okay with the fact I couldn't say his name. He attributed it to the brain damage. But later, when I did make a few garbled attempts, I could see his eyes glaze over and I knew that I had hurt him. By trying to say his name, I had hurt him. No, I can compensate. We will talk without names. Gretch takes a deep breath and continues.

"How long has it been?" Gretch's voice remains determined as she slowly lists the months on her fingers. "February, March, April, May, June, July."

I listen, very aware of where she's headed with all this. I want to tell her to back off, but I just lower my head like a disobedient child.

"You know you could say his name if you wanted to."

I shake my head defiantly. "Can't."

"It's been six months, Becki. You hear his name over and over every day."

"Can't," I repeat, studying the thin sheets of steel on the bleachers beneath my feet. "Can't."

Then Gretch turns to me, this sister who knows all my secrets, my links to the past, and is able to see right through me.

"You could say Denny, Den, or Dennis. You COULD say it."

"Can't." I shake her off and deny it. "Can't. Can't." Gretch shrugs her shoulders and looks away.

"Okay, whatever. If you can't, you can't." Gretch begins to speak faster and faster and it makes my head spin. I try to concentrate on the words pouring from her lips.

"But tell me why you can't say Denny. Tell me, tell me, tell me," she says over and over again.

"Tell me...."

I can't stand it. She's like a movie on fast-forward. I cover my ears and shout, "Can't say Den!"

Gretch smiles. She won; she gets her way. But I win too. I grab her arm and now it's my turn to talk fast, afraid it might slip away if I stop.

"Den, Den-nis, Den-ny," I say breaking the word into its parts. A rush of adrenalin takes over my body and I'm laughing and crying and screaming—now to Denny. "Den, Den, DENNY!"

DENNY

After almost six long months of waiting, she finally says it. My mouth drops open and the racket slips from my hand as I move toward her, legs running, arms pumping, until our eyes lock and she's whispering now, "Den."

It's the sweetest sound I've ever heard. I'm no fool, I know we have a long way to go yet, but I feel like I have my Bec back; I have us back. Soon we're ambushed by Gretch and Jim, all of us crying and laughing as Becki repeats my name over and over, "Den, Denny, Dennis."

NEBRASKA!?

BECKI

Nebraska? Where the heck is Nebraska? What—is a Nebraska?

Denny tells me he got a letter from the University of Nebraska asking him to come for a job interview. The job would be in a small town in northeast Nebraska named Norfolk, where he would be a hydrogeologist with the geological survey part of the university.

What is a Norfolk? Why can't he find a job closer to Mom and Dad's home? He has an offer in a small town about 15 miles away, but they want to ship him to New Mexico for three to four months right away, so he doesn't think that is the best thing for a family trying to start over again.

Well, I guess we will just need to take a day at a time, a step at a time, and see what the Lord has in store for us. Little do I know how much I will be learning about corn and canning and Big Red football!

THE CAT SCAN

BECKI

There's no way I can fake this. This CAT scan has to prove that there are no more ruptures or aneurysms in the blood vessels in my brain. If there is any sign of another aneurysm, we can't move to Nebraska for Denny's new position as a hydrogeologist. So, this is a big deal.

Dr. Becker first tells us that a CAT (computerized axial tomography) scan is a relatively new technology and that they have only had the machine about two months. I am one of the first people to get a CAT scan in the Milwaukee area. Like an obedient student nervous about a final, I lie back on the crisp white paper lining the patient table.

I look through the opening of the encasement covering me and feel a little like Snow White in her glass coffin. After a few more excruciating minutes, a technician nods at Dr. Becker and I know it's time to begin.

A wave of anxiety rushes through my whole body. I can feel the sweat trickle down the side of my forehead but I can't move my arms to brush it away. Is it supposed to be this hot in here? I'm burning up, but I have to make it through this. I have to pass.

As my breathing becomes more rapid, I lose control and begin to cry. I can't do this. Thankfully, Dr. Becker distracts me by knocking on the window. He smiles warmly at me and gives me a thumbs up, whispering, "It'll be okay."

Denny is behind him and nods in agreement. Their strength is so comforting I can feel the tension leave my body as I begin to relax.

"Okay Becki, try not to move," Dr. Becker says as the machine clicks away, first to my right, then to the top of my head, click, then to my left, click, feeding information to the computer next to it. Finally, after about fifteen minutes, the CAT scan is over.

Afterwards, Dr. Becker tells us he'll call with the results as soon as he has them. Next, it's Denny's turn for his test—finishing the first draft of his thesis.

And if all goes well for us, we'll be on our way and on our own in Nebraska.

THE OUTING

BECKI

After the CAT scan, Denny has to get to school to talk to his advisor about his thesis, so he drops me off at Lynn's place, which is in the same apartment building we live in.

Lynn and I were dormmates at Valparaiso University and now she's on her way to a master's degree in sociology at the University of Wisconsin–Milwaukee. She was also my confidante when I first drunkenly admitted I was in love with Denny. It was after my third date with Denny that I plopped down on my bed and exclaimed, "I love him!"

Lynn laughed and shook her head, "You're just drunk. You can't be in love this fast."

But I knew I was. I looked at Lynn, who was usually the serious one, and in a most determined manner I shook my head and repeated the words, "I love him."

Now, five years later, my earlier revelation proving true, Lynn and I are again dormmates for the day.

"So, how'd it go?" Lynn asks.

I shrug my shoulders. "We'll know soon enough."

Since we both have errands to run before Denny returns, we buckle Aimee in the back seat of Lynn's old Ford Pinto and head for the store. Aimee needs juice and I need supplies for dinner tonight.

It is a typical August afternoon, hot and muggy except for the occasional breeze that floats in off of Lake Michigan. Lynn starts rolling her window down and motions for me to do the same. "Whew, that's a little better," she says and shoves the key in the ignition.

As we drive through the city, the heat becomes more and more unbearable. Aimee begins crying in the back seat as hot air blasts her from both sides, but since there is no air conditioning, we can't close the windows for fear of overheating even more. The heat makes me feel clammy and dizzy, so dizzy I can't look out the window. Everything begins spinning around me so I close my eyes and try to fight off the inevitable car sickness.

"You alright?" Lynn asks, but her voice drowns in Aimee's screams and I can't answer.

LYNN

I thought Becki was just getting car sick but when her body starts shaking violently, I know she is having a grand mal seizure. I chastise myself for not asking Denny what to do if this happens.

Becki's legs kick out and while I try to restrain her with one hand, I maneuver the car to a stop with the other. All the while, Aimee screams in discomfort. I try my most soothing voice, but to no avail.

"There, there Aimee. There, there."

I stop abruptly in the parking lot of the convenience store and run inside. Aimee continues to scream, but I have to get help for Becki first.

"Can I use the phone?" I ask, trying to catch my breath. "My friend just had a grand mal seizure."

The young clerk looks at me apologetically and explains, "Sorry, it's not for public use."

I stand for a moment in disbelief. Maybe she didn't hear me correctly, or doesn't understand. "Do you get what I'm telling you? My friend just had a grand mal seizure."

"Sorry," the clerk repeats, "There's a pay phone outside." Now I am infuriated. If this girl thinks I am going to go any farther for a phone, she's nuts.

"Listen," I snarl at her in a voice I will never admit was my own, enunciating every word in a threatening manner, I say again, "Give me the damned phone. My friend had a grand mal seizure."

The clerk's eyes grow wide, but she doesn't budge. She seems frozen in place, whether out of fear or curiosity, I'm not sure. All I know is that I can't waste any more time on her. I jump over the counter and grab the phone. The girl steps back, probably thinking I am a maniac, but I don't care. I call the police.

I almost feel bad for scaring her. Almost. "Dumb rule," I mumble as I run out to check on Becki and Aimee. Within minutes, an ambulance arrives. Poor Aimee is still inconsolable as I rock her in my arms and watch the EMT team place Becki in the ambulance and turn the sirens on. Aimee screams even louder as they speed away.

BECKI

I'm so tired. That's one of the side effects of a grand mal seizure. When you wake up, you feel like gravity's doing a number on you. Every muscle in my body feels weighed down, and I think I could probably sleep a full day if they'd let me. But I can't. I'm in the hospital again. I groan and rub my eyes.

Gotta' get outa' here, I think. Then I see Denny sitting next to me.

"You're okay, Bec," he says. "You just decided to add a little more excitement to our lives with a grand mal seizure." This was the first seizure I had since the rupture on February 1st.

"Lynn and Aimee, okay?"

"Yeah, don't worry. Lynn said she'll watch Aimee as long as we need her."

Our plans, I thought. What about Nebraska?

I don't want to ask Denny because I am afraid of what he might say. Because of me, our plans are ruined again. I look down at the white sheet resting on my stomach. Is this all I can expect? Seizures and hospital beds for the rest of my life?

"Hey," Denny whispers, lifting my face to his. "You're not staying. The doctor said it was a post-operative seizure due to healing of scar tissue and everything else looks good. You're still healing, Bec.

"Nebraska?" I ask.

Denny grins. "Nebraska's on.

VELDA

I know I shouldn't be saying this, but I can't help it. I think Denny's gone nuts. Nebraska?

I can understand Becki being okay with this because her processing abilities have gone through some changes. But Denny? I just can't believe it. He is taking her to Nebraska. Nine hours from her family! I've been working with her, trying to help her regain her language and motor skills. I've been trying to get her to be able to take care of herself, but I'm not sure she is ready to be on her own yet. Granted, she'll have Denny, but he'll be working for the university, and Becki will be left alone during the day to care for Aimee. This is just too scary for me to even think about.

* * *

When Becki first got out of the hospital, I took a leave from my job so I could help her regain her independence. I thought I'd have more time to get my daughter back to her old sassy, confident self. Now I know that isn't in the cards, at least for a while.

I need help so I take Becki to a neurologist hoping for some advice, maybe new techniques that might help her be more successful. Maybe the doctor can suggest a good speech therapist. But the only thing he suggests is that rehabilitation is futile.

Basically, "What you see is what you get." He says, "Becki belongs in an institution to fill her days. His words are so harsh and matter-of-fact, they sting!

I can't bear it. Becki looks like someone has knocked the wind right out of her. So as cool as I can muster, I look him up and down like the pathetic idiot he was when he made his proclamation and say, "I hope that isn't true, doctor, because if that is what you really think, then you're just a pompous, balding idiot who has no idea what my daughter is capable of." Now it is his turn to look deflated.

I take Becki's arm and we walk out without saying another word. The door closes behind us. In the silence, I pray for my daughter. I pray for her future. And I pray she will be ready for Nebraska.

That visit continues to bother me. There's more to Becki than what that doctor saw. But I also realize Becki is not ready for all the responsibilities she'll have when she leaves. So, it may sound harsh, but I can't help thinking Denny has gone nuts.

Gratefully, my thoughts are interrupted by Becki's call for help. "Aimee's got more applesauce on herself and her mother than in her mouth."

MY SPECIAL SPEECH THERAPIST

BECKI

Although I'm not having formal therapy this summer, other than Mom keeping my nose to the grindstone, I do have my own special speech therapist come and help me all summer. My dearest friend since kindergarten, Becky, is a speech pathologist. She received her master's degree a year ago and worked in a school district this past year not far from Elgin, where she also lives. Becky also came to see me while I was still in the hospital, so she knows what she has in store for her. She comes to help me two days each week.

Today, when she gets here, I am having trouble saying "breakfast." I struggle each day trying to tell Mom what I want first thing in the morning, and I am still having trouble asking for breakfast. Becky is trying all sorts of tricks as I try to read the word written on a piece of paper. All I can seem to come up with is "brickfiss," or "brack fass," or "break fake." Becky then writes down *brk fst* on the piece of paper. Right away, I look at it and say exactly those sounds and it comes out as "breakfast." I guess those vowels they stick in words really mess me up.

I am so happy and thankful to have my dearest friend, who knows what I used to be able to do, help me learn how to speak again. I don't have to worry about being embarrassed around her. She has helped me a lot and I really love her for it.

BECKY (BECKI'S DEAREST FRIEND)

Was I ever in for a reality check! After receiving my master's degree in speech pathology and working for a year in the schools, I thought I knew pretty much everything there was to know about speech therapy. But after working with Becki this summer, I realize there is still a lot I don't know. Nothing in school could have prepared me to be face to face with my good friend since kindergarten, who is now 24 years old and struggles to communicate. I think I helped her quite a bit, but boy, did she ever help me as well. This has certainly been an experience I won't forget.

CHAPTER 5

THE NEXT LEG OF THE JOURNEY ON OUR OWN

SEPTEMBER 1976—THE TRIP TO NORFOLK

DENNY

Today's the day. Becki's dad, Cal, and I pack up the U-Haul truck with all our belongings that were gathering dust in storage, while Velda helps Becki and Aimee pack up the other two cars.

Three hours later, the U-Haul is crammed with furniture, lamps, and boxes piled on top of each other. The two cars look no better, and I can see the weight of it all has caused the bodies of the cars to sink lower into the tires. They're bursting to the windows with blankets, baby items, and all the other small necessities we can't fit in the U-Haul. But we're on a mission. This will take one trip and one trip only.

Next stop, the apartment I found for us in Norfolk. I check things over one last time to make sure I haven't forgotten anything before we leave. Nothing here.

The place in Nebraska will be more like home. The new place will be ours—Bec, me, and Aimee—a fresh start. It's an old green three-story house with high ceilings and spacious rooms. We have the main floor, and I know Bec's going to love the kitchen filled with windows taking in the sunrise. Only thing is, it will be just the three of us.

There will be no parents or friends to turn to in a pinch. We don't know a single person in Norfolk. A moment of self-doubt hits me. Maybe Velda is right. Maybe we are crazy.

Enough of that! So, what if we are, I tell myself. It's time we move on. Becki and I both agree we need to move on with our lives and start earning some money, and this job is perfect. I have an office in Norfolk so I can be close to home, with only monthly trips to the University in Lincoln. Becki will have a little bit of independence, but I'll still be close by if she needs me.

I leave the key on the kitchen counter of my friend's apartment where I had stayed the last couple of months and head back downstairs.

"Ready!" Cal nods back at me and gets into his blue Chevy station wagon while Velda, Becki, and Aimee climb into our little cream-colored Nova.

"Follow me," I tell them, climbing into the U-Haul. Crazy or not, here we go.

BECKI

The drive to Norfolk seems like a hazy dream. The sound of the engine lulls me to sleep, and I don't wake up until we are on the highway staring at a stretch of cornfields dotted with gas stations and rest stops here and there. It's been about two hours now, our prearranged time limit before we stop. I need to take my Dilantin, and Aimee needs to get out of the car for a while. Denny sees another rest stop and pulls in.

Taking medications isn't my favorite thing to do, especially because it makes me so tired, but it's supposed to control the seizures. Mom hands me the pills and leads me to the water fountain. She looks a bit frazzled. (She doesn't have any pills to make her sleep through the trip.) Not wanting to miss an opportunity to lighten the situation, I tease her a bit. "You drug me to sleep for trip, Mom?"

Mom shakes her head. "Oh, Becki, don't be silly!" Not one to be outdone in the teasing department, she adds, "You know I'd only do that to your father!"

Denny, having a built-in time clock, taps his watch, and waves us back. He closes the door on the U-Haul, then makes sure we're all accounted for. Dad opens the car doors and we scoot back to our seats, ready for the road again.

HOME AT LAST!

BECKI

This place is amazing! There's so much space compared to our first two apartments in Valpo and Milwaukee, and well, it's been tight at my parent's home with all of us there, so this is like moving into a mansion. I even have a dining room with a wall of mirrors right off the kitchen. Separate rooms! Our old apartment had the kitchen, dining room, and living room all wrapped into one area.

Denny takes us on a tour, and everything's looking great until we get to the bathroom. I look at Mom, because she is a nurse, I know she has a thing about sterile bathrooms. This one is far from sterile.

"Out," she warns us. "Looks like this room hasn't seen a disinfectant in ages. I'll just clean up a little first."

Dad and I exchange looks. We know Mom never cleans up a little. She tears everything apart, power washes, boils anything she can lift, and wipes down everything else!

I shrug and motion to Denny to get out of Mom's way. She's putting her plastic gloves on, a definite sign that germs are gonna fly. Sure enough, the first thing Mom does is rip out the furry pink carpeting, bags it, and immediately carries it out of the apartment at arm's length. Then she's spraying disinfectants, scrubbing, steaming, and boiling everything in sight. It's quite a show.

The men get bored, though, and leave Aimee and me to watch while they unload the vehicles. After every germ has been destroyed, Mom tells Dad to take Denny to pick up new vinyl flooring, which she then installs for the finishing touches. Voilà, we have a new bathroom!

ANOTHER OPTIMISTIC DOCTOR

BECKI

Denny set up an appointment with a neurosurgeon in Lincoln for the Monday after we arrive in Norfolk so that Mom and Dad can go along with us. Although we will have a family doctor in Norfolk for my meds, Denny and I think it is a good idea to have a neurosurgeon on board to help me continue with my rehabilitation.

Boy! We thought the neurosurgeon we saw in Elgin had the personality of a rock. This new guy must be related because he isn't much better. He tells us again, "What you see is what you get."

He doesn't give me much hope for regaining more of my abilities or give me ideas on what I can do next. Well, it doesn't take us long to decide that this isn't the guy we want to help me get my life back on track. I guess we had been spoiled by Dr. Uttech, who along with his fantastic surgical skills, also had a great personality.

DENNY

In all fairness to the profession of neurosurgery, I think we start to realize that these men are excellent, well-respected surgeons who daily deal with some of the gravest life-threatening situations, but what happens beyond the operating room is not necessarily their forte.

Their jobs are to save lives. We need to turn to other professionals to help Becki regain her abilities. We eventually find a neurologist (not a neurosurgeon) in Lincoln who is very helpful, and optimistic, in mapping out our next steps.

THREE DAYS LATER

BECKI

I know I wanted to move out here, but I didn't realize how hard it would be to say good-bye to my parents. Denny and I settle into the apartment with Aimee. Everything's put away, and now it's time for Mom and Dad to drive back home.

They've played such an integral part in my healing to this point, made me feel safe when I was scared, and understood me when I couldn't get the words out. I know I can't express how much I appreciate what they've done for me, for us, or how deeply I feel about them so I just say, "I love you," and hope it's enough.

Dad hugs us and loads their suitcases in the car. "Call if you need anything!"

Mom kisses Aimee and Denny, then hugs me. "We love you too, baby." Her eyes are brimming with tears, and she hesitates for a moment.

I nod at her and smile. "It's okay."

"Yes." She smiles back and, almost as if she's forcing her feet to move, she turns around and gets in the car.

And then they're gone.

Unsure about starting over without my parents, I lean against Denny. God has just handed me my second chance at life. What an amazing but scary gift. I hope I don't blow it.

Little do we know the roles our neighbors and the people at our new church, Christ Lutheran, will play in our next steps to recovery. And then there are also Frank and Helen, who live in Lincoln.

Frank is Denny's co-worker at the university. He and his wife Helen become our surrogate parents and grandparents. When we take trips to Lincoln, Denny drops me off at their house, where Aimee and I stay while Denny is at work. They are just wonderful, loving, and caring people, always ready to help out. Helen even watches Aimee while I take a nap, since I can still get overtired at times. And Frank is always thinking of things that Denny might need help with.

Once, when we were heading back to Norfolk, Frank asks Denny if he wants to check the oil in the car before we take off. Denny couldn't figure out why the heck Frank would even ask that because it seems kind of out of the blue, but he thought why not. When Frank checked the oil, the dipstick didn't have anything on it. We consider Frank and Helen our guardian angels!

NOVEMBER 3, 1976—THE BIRTHDAY CAKE

BECKI

Aimee turns one today! I can't believe it's already been a year. She's grown so much; she's even talking a little and calling me Momma. I figure if she keeps it up, she'll surpass me in the speech department. (Which may just happen because we haven't been able to find a therapist to help me with my speech yet.) But I won't think about that now.

I have a birthday cake to make. Since Aimee loves angel food cake, I bought a cake mix, compliments of Betty Crocker, and I'm feeling a bit like the happy homemaker as I look at the box and try to figure out what I need.

"First get bowl," I tell myself. I have a picture in my head of all the items I need, and I remember that they're under the counter. I bend down and pull out a bowl. Then get the beater and a pan.

Aimee is walking around the kitchen, opening up drawers, and glancing at me every once in a while, as I start talking myself through each step. This is supposed to be her naptime but, of course, she's not tired today. I turn the whole experience into a cooking show.

"This is a bowl," I tell Aimee and sit her down in front of me.

"And this is a…..," a what? I ask myself looking at the contraption with its white handle and silver slotted thingamajigs.

The word *beater* is lost somewhere in my brain, so I make up a word. "It is a *hernzebekana*. It mixes the stuff up. See?"

I wave it in the air and turn the handle. "Whirr, whirr!" Aimee squeals with delight and reaches for the beater. "No, no. Owie," I tell her and give her one of her toys instead.

Now where was I? Oh yeah, measuring cups. After I get those out of the drawer, I look at my directions again.

"Put……m-m-m-mix in bo-oo-wl. A-d-d one c-u-p w-at-er." I sound out every letter. Then I look at my bowl. Now what did that direction say? I have to look at the box again. This time, I stop after each sentence and do what it says before I forget again. After about an hour of this, I finally have my cake mix ready to be beaten.

I grab the beater, but just my luck, I can't remember how to use the damned thing. Well, I'll just plug it in and play with the buttons until I figure it out. Once it starts whirring, I lower it into the bowl. Cake mix flies everywhere. I'll have to remember for next time to put the beater in the bowl before turning it on. Then it whirs and clanks on the sides until I can smooth out my hand movements. Finally, I get it.

Aimee claps her hands in appreciation of the noise. I smile at her. The struggle to make this cake is worth it. Aimee is having a grand time. Now the cake's ready for the oven. I pour it into the pan.

"Pan," I tell Aimee pointing to it. Aimee forms the sound with her lips. "Ppppppp." As I practice saying the words on the box, I'm also teaching Aimee in my own awkward way how to speak.

"Now we put it in the oven," I tell her. I check the temperature. 350 degrees. "Ready." I put the pan in the oven and set the timer. After the whole process is complete, my cake is ready to be frosted, and it only took three hours, a floor full of pans, and a blanket of white dust on my counters. No matter, I did it all by myself. To really make it special, I spread green frosting on top to match her birthday present: a green winter coat.

If I may say so myself, it's lovely.

DENNY

When I came home for lunch today, Bec was struggling to read the directions for Aimee's cake. I wasn't sure what I would find when I got home after work, but to my surprise, we have a wonderful angel food cake cooling on the counter. After dinner, Bec brings out the cake.

The look on her face is priceless. At first, I wasn't sure if she should go through the frustration of trying to make this cake, but now I'm glad she did. When she sets it on the table, she is absolutely beaming with pride. And when Aimee shoves a handful in her mouth and says, "More," Bec kisses her frosting-covered cheeks and puts another piece on her tray. I get the next piece of cake and a frosting kiss from Bec. She smears it on my lips, and laughs, admiring her work.

That's when I know things are really going to be okay. The aneurysm and the medications, and everything else Bec went through aren't going to take her spark away. Her confidence is growing, and she is on her way back.

BECKI

I'm exhausted. Making that birthday cake has shown me a couple of things. For one, I'm a terrible reader. And that hurts a bit, me with an English degree and all. I used to love reading, loved analyzing language, but now I see that isn't possible anymore. It took a lot out of me to read each direction on that cake mix box, but I have to remember that just a few months ago, I wouldn't have been able to read a single line. This time, I read the whole thing. Granted it took me hours to do so, but I didn't give up and I had a satisfied birthday girl to show for it.

Second, I have to give myself a break. I was getting a bit frustrated when I kept forgetting the instructions and had to read them all over again. No matter how painful it is to admit, I realize I'm not the same girl I was a year ago. And I may never be able to do all the things that once came so easily to me.

As I lie in bed and ponder these thoughts, Denny walks in with weights in both hands in nothing more than his jockeys. He begins exercising, lifting the weights and bending his legs, up down, up down. And although I haven't seen him do this since before I went to the hospital, I remember his routine. It's both comical and sexy at the same time.

I watch him and a warm feeling washes over me, and I realize how much I love him. This is my Denny, content with his life, our life, exercising before bed. Physically, I'm drained, but maybe I have a little energy left for Denny. And emotionally, I'm ready. The aneurysm has left me feeling disconnected to the most important relationship in my life, my husband. And with all the changes, Denny could've said it was too much and left. Instead, he fought for me. He fought for us.

Now, watching my husband lift his weights in his underwear seems the most natural thing to do. I feel connected to him again, comfortable with him, and more in love than ever.

"Denny," I say and reach for his hand.

He puts down his weights and joins me at the edge of the bed. "Huh?

"Let's…"

He looks puzzled, unsteady. It reminds me of our first time.

"Are you sure?"

"More sure of this than anything else." I sit up and wrap my arms around him.

"But what if…"

Always the scientist, thinking facts and the hypothesis and results of too much pressure on my brain. I can almost see all the thoughts racing through his head, and I just want to wipe them away.

We made love the night before I had my aneurysm and I went into a coma. He doesn't want to hurt me.

"Shhh," I whisper. "I'll be okay." Then I see the tension drain from his face and I know he's not thinking like a scientist anymore; he's thinking like the man I made love to so many times before. He pulls me closer, and we sink into bed slowly, softly making love.

FEBRUARY 1977—OUCH, MY FINGER!

DENNY

Becki's mom and dad are here visiting us. We are just getting ready to go to church on Sunday morning when all of a sudden

Bec starts to feel funny. Before we know it, she is down on the floor flailing and wailing. She is having a grand mal seizure again. She hasn't had one since we were back in Milwaukee.

Boy, do I get a rude awakening! I now know that it is actually a myth that when someone is having a grand mal seizure, you should stick something between their teeth to keep them from swallowing their tongue.

Well, the closest thing I have to use is my finger. Ouch!! Boy, does she clamp down hard. Fortunately, I am able to get my finger out while it is still attached, although with a nice big tooth mark.

Bec has another seizure a couple months later. The doctor checks her blood chemistry levels and in addition to taking Dilantin, he puts her on phenobarbital. I guess this is a reminder that we never know for sure what lies ahead of us.

SUMMER 1977—OUR FIRST REAL "HOME SWEET HOME"

BECKI

After searching for months, we buy our first home in a quiet little subdivision on the edge of Norfolk. It is our first big investment.

The house has a beautiful backyard and there are other neatly maintained homes nestled along the street. Best yet, it's only a few blocks from the grocery store and from our church. The only problem, as I see it is, I don't know anyone. But, if I can count on my wits, that won't be a problem for long.

I work on my conversation skills with Denny, and then practice it on my neighbors. Hopefully, we have nice neighbors and my slow speech won't scare them away. So, for the next few days, Aimee and I play outside and, according to plan, I meet all my neighbors.

THE CANNING QUEEN

BECKI

It seems like everyone in Norfolk cans—fruits and vegetables— that is. There are canned beets, canned beans, canned corn, canned tomatoes, and canned peaches. You name it, someone in Norfolk probably cans it and sells it at the local farmer's market.

I eventually learn to can too, but not without some resistance. Learning to can opens new doors for me. I focus more on my family's eating habits. But almost as important, I make a very dear friend, Lucy, the canning queen.

Lucy is the first neighbor to walk over and introduce herself. She is a grandma and a cook at the local Catholic school.

Since meeting Lucy, we've become pretty good friends. She listens patiently when we talk about our kids, or when I'm struggling with a particular word. Maybe it's because she has a child with a disability that she is so understanding. Or maybe she's one of the few people, besides my family, who can see past my disability and know me for who I really am. Whatever it is, I'm grateful for our newfound friendship. She introduces me to the world of home food processing and canning.

"You should prepare fresh vegetables for Aimee. It's healthier," she tells me. Within an afternoon's time, I learn how to whip up an exceptionally good vegetable puree that can also be used as finger paint, especially the beets.

Next, I learn how to process food to store through the winter. Gosh, I'm starting to feel like a pilgrim. "That's what stores are for, you know. All you have to do is fill up your cart and go. *Voilà!* You don't have to boil all these bottles."

Lucy just laughs and hands me a bowl full of peaches. "You're in Nebraska now, my dear. This is what you do, you put up!"

"You put up?" I look at her quizzically.

"Yeah, you put up," she explains.

I'm still not getting it.

"Put up! You know, can the vegetables."

The light goes on. "Oh." I take a few minutes to process the phrase. "So, if you put them up, do they get heavy? Do you have to put them down, then?"

Lucy shakes her head and giggles. "Very funny."

I love hearing Lucy laugh. We kid around like two young girls without a care in the world, canning to our hearts' content. And I can forget about my problems, even if it's just for a few hours.

We spend the afternoon canning peaches, beans, corn, and the dust bunnies under the table. You name it, we canned it. And let me tell you, it's a much more involved process than making baby food. There are all these rules. The temperature has to be just right. It has to be sealed perfectly or it could spoil.

Then Lucy says, "If we don't seal it tight, you could get botulism." Sounds bad, so I'm very careful to follow all Lucy's instructions.

Still, when I'm done, I think I'll try it out on Denny first. If it kills him, then I'll know not to give any to Aimee.

* * *

Feeling a bit adventurous, I walk to the Hinky Dinky grocery store (I love to say that name, it kinda flows, like *hernzebekana*) and buy six crates of Colorado peaches for $15. Some are rotten but most are okay. Then, with the assistance of my little helper, Aimee, I can thirty-five quarts of peaches and make a pretty tasty peach syrup too.

When Denny comes home, he can't believe his eyes. It looks like Hinky Dinky has moved the store to our counter.

"You did this?

Before I can say anything, Aimee puts her sticky hands on her hips. She has glistening streaks of wild hair where she has run her fingers through during our mushing and mixing of the peaches, and she is indignant.

"Daddy, we did it ALL." I have to laugh. Needless to say, we eat peaches for two years straight.

THE WORKOUTS

BECKI

Denny's having a hard time finding a speech therapist in Norfolk for me. He started his search on a wider scale, but in the meantime, he sets up a physical therapy routine for me. Every night after he gets home from work, I must run. Denny lays out the path for me: three times around the block is a mile. His instructions are specific.

"Becki," he says. "Go up to the corner and follow the sidewalk around. You keep going until you come back around the corner to us. DO NOT CROSS THE STREET!"

I nod and begin my jogging excursion with my audience, Denny and Aimee, cheering me on. Aimee is developing her speech and mimics Denny.

"Go, Mommy! Good, Mommy!" or "More, Mommy!" She is so happy to see me come around the corner each time, clapping and yelling to me, that I feel like I am running in the Olympics. At first, I can only make half the length of one lap, but after a few weeks, I am up to a mile.

My coordination continues to be poor, but I am getting faster. Finally, after about two months, my arms pump in time with the movements of my legs. I am ready for more.

JANUARY 1978—
SCHOOL DAYS: BACK TO FOURTH GRADE

BECKI

Denny has given me quite a few challenges lately. Last Friday, I tackled all the grocery shopping while Denny and Aimee walked behind. He says he wants me to read the list and find the items myself. Part of me, though, thinks Denny's just trying to get out of doing the work. I read his lists all day. He has a list of chores for me to do around the house. He has a list detailing Aimee's schedule, and he has a list of exercises I can do in between.

The lists have improved my reading ability, but I still have to sound out bigger words. That's when I come up with the idea to go back to school. But where? I can't go back to college; those books will seem like a foreign language, and my writing consists of chicken scratches and smaller words, and that's on a good day.

No, I will definitely bomb in college. But what if I go back to grade school? Maybe fourth grade? I loved fourth grade; I was smart in fourth grade. And now, it might be just enough of a challenge to help me improve my reading skills without being too overwhelming.

I know it's crazy, but I have to give it a try. I want to be able to read more than a list. I want to read books to my daughter, not just tell her the story from memory. I want to read the newspaper again, not just look at the pictures. I want to know the things I used to know, and if going back to fourth grade could help me get it, I'll sit in a little desk with nine- and ten-year-olds and raise my hand just like the rest of them.

DENNY

She says my lists are tough, yet she wants to go back to school. I'm not going to discourage her, though, because I think it just might work. I still haven't been able to locate a speech therapist for her, so this is the next best thing. We're good friends with the pastor and family at our church and the principal and his family at our parochial grade school, and I'm pretty sure they'll help us out and let Becki sit in a few of the classes at the school.

BECKI

I am a little nervous about asking Pastor Karl if I can join the fourth graders at Christ Lutheran Grade School, but he is so nice about it. We set up a schedule where I go twice a week for the reading and language arts class, and Aimee stays with Pastor Karl's wife, Rhoda.

They have a little girl Aimee's age so it works out perfectly. This will be the first time I leave Aimee with anyone else besides my parents or Mrs. T. Hope she'll do okay.

Oh, yeah—Who is Mrs T? Mrs. T is an elderly lady in our congregation who loves to babysit little children. Some friends referred her to us, and we also see her every Sunday morning at church and in Bible study. Aimee always likes to go and sit on her lap during Bible study.

If you were ever asked to describe the sweetest, most gracious, and caring person you know, it would be Mrs. T. She does not always accept payment because she considers herself honored for us to ask her to babysit Aimee. Wow! So we make sure we find other ways to provide her the compensation she deserves. Mrs. T is truly one of those great blessings in life that we will never forget. She understands my situation and limitations very well. She is a very important part of my journey and my road back!

THE NEW KID

BECKI

I feel as nervous as I did when it actually was my first day at school. I drop Aimee off at Pastor Karl's house, and his wife, Rhoda, greets me at the door.

"Hi, Becki! Hi, Aimee!" she says and motions us to come in.

"I have a little girl who can't wait to play," she laughs. Then her daughter Gretchen, who's about two, runs over to Aimee and leads her to the toys. I relax a bit as my little girl runs off like a princess in a castle, enjoying her new playmate.

Rhoda winks at me. "Don't worry, we'll take good care of her."

"I know," I say, wishing Aimee would have at least hugged me goodbye. But she's my little independent Aimee, not afraid of anything. I wish I could say the same about me. Maybe this isn't such a good idea after all. What am I thinking? Maybe I should just forget the whole thing. Rhoda's pretty nice. Maybe I'll just stay and chat with her.

Rhoda doesn't let me, though. "You'd better go, Becki. Mrs. Larsen is expecting you. It'll be fine!" she reminds me.

Well, stalling is out, so I walk over to the school. It's a beautiful brick building with children's' artwork peeking out of the windows. Inside, the halls are quiet, but as I pass each room, I can hear the bustle of children moving, little voices, giggling and talking, and adult voices giving directions and guiding the students into the next activity.

I need to find room 21.

Denny and Pastor Karl walked me through these halls last week, so I'm pretty sure I'm heading in the right direction. I look on the doors. Yep, 17, 19, on the right, 21 is next. The door is open and I see a row of desks lined neatly in front of one another. The room is quiet except for the sound of whispers and Mrs. Larsen's voice.

"Everyone, get out your vocabulary books. We'll start chapter three today."

She sounds nice. I take a step closer and peek in a bit. The kids look harmless. This might not be so bad after all.

Mrs. Larsen sees me. "Come in, Mrs. Lawton. We've been hoping you'd join us!"

"Thank you," I say and walk in.

Mrs. Larsen shows me to my desk. Since I'm the tallest fourth grader, it's in the back of the room. I squeeze myself into my desk and lean back. Luckily, the wall is right behind me and gives me a little more support. Then she has each of the students introduce themselves. Afterward, she introduces me.

"This is Mrs. Lawton. She'll be joining us every Tuesday and Thursday for reading and language arts class."

I raise my hand. "Mrs. Larsen?"

"Yes?"

"I'm a student." I say as respectfully as I can. (I don't want her to think I'm a troublemaker my very first day.) "Please call me Becki."

Mrs. Larsen smiles. "All right." She hands me a reading book, along with a vocabulary workbook. "Becki it is."

I look at the faces around me. They're smiling, too.

Mrs. Larsen begins writing words on the board. "Right now, we're copying the words in our workbook, Becki." She looks at the boy next to me. "Mike, show Becki where to write the words." Mike nods and points to where I should begin.

"Thanks," I say and press the page down. Mike goes back to his writing. I pick up my pencil and try to form the first word she prints on the board. f a l l. I'm not sure what the word is yet. I'll worry about sounding it out later. For now, I'll concentrate on placing letters on the page. I press the pencil into the paper and accidentally chip a little piece off. Oh well, I don't want to interrupt the class again, so I just keep working. The letters look odd, like they had been written by a child instead of a grown woman of 25.

F a l l. Finished.

I look over at Mike's page. He's at least five words ahead of me. This is humiliating. I can't let anyone see I'm only on the second word. I hunch forward and begin the next word. Winter. W I ...

"Okay, everyone, let's sound out the words."

Sound out the words? I haven't even written them down yet.

"Lisa, try the first one." She points at the word. It looks tough. Silently, I try to piece the letters together into a coherent word.

I almost have all the letters together when Lisa answers, "Fall."

"Good." Mrs. Larsen looks around the room. Most of the children are waving their hands in the air, hoping to be called on. I raise my hand slowly. I'm not sure I want her to call on me. I might get it wrong and look stupid. The kids might even laugh at me. *Stop it*, I tell myself. You're a grown woman. Do you want to be able to read again or not? I wave my hand in the air just as vigorously as the rest of the class.

Mrs. Larsen nods at me. "Becki, read the next one, please." She points to winter.

"W—www-i-i-wwwii-wwiinn..." Making the n and t come together is proving very difficult. Mrs. Larsen waits patiently for me to sound it out. Everyone else is waiting too, they probably haven't seen anyone struggle like this since first grade. I'm starting to feel a little self-conscious. "Win-Winnn-t...

Mike leans over. "Winter," he whispers.

That's it! "Winter!" I shout, triumphantly, glad the word is finally out.

"Right!" says Mrs. Larsen and everyone claps. I smile at Mike and whisper back, "Thank you." He smiles back at me. I guess angels come in all sizes.

STORY TIME

BECKI

"And then Goldilocks eats the porridge and gets tired. Daddy bear's bed is too hard. Momma bear's bed is too soft, but Baby bear's bed is just right."

"No, Mommy," Aimee informs me. "Read it right."

I can see faking it isn't going to get me anywhere anymore. *Goldilocks and the Three Bears* is Aimee's favorite bedtime story. Denny has read it to her so many times that she has most of it memorized. I'm going to have to pick stories Aimee isn't familiar with.

Hopefully, soon I'll be able to read ALL the words in Aimee's books. I want to read to her so badly. I sit with Aimee and Denny when he reads to her, watching the way he animates the story with his voice and how Aimee becomes more and more entranced. She can hardly wait for him to turn the page.

I want to read stories like that. I want Aimee to look forward to story time with me, too. I can tell she would rather have Denny read to her. He reads so smoothly. I read a few of the words and have to make up the rest. Now, Aimee's getting wise to my game.

All I need is a little more time. I'm getting better at sounding out the tougher words, thanks to Mrs. Larsen's class. And my sight vocabulary has increased, too. I may never read like Denny, maybe not even as well as those wonderful fourth graders, but hopefully, I will read. That's all I need right now.

SUMMER 1978 — THE BABY BLUES

BECKI

Denny and I have been talking about having another child. I know it sounds crazy, but we've always wanted two. And I think I can handle it now. It's been just over two years since I had my aneurysm, and I'm much stronger now. Sure, I'm a little dented – literally, on the left side of my head – and bruised, but I think I'm functioning pretty well.

Case in point, Denny doesn't have to write schedules or lists for me anymore. I can read enough to get by, and although my word retrieval is still poor, I'm now able to express myself so others understand. I can hold my own in an adult conversation.

I drive our car. Even though I haven't had a seizure for over a year and I got my driver's license again, Denny prefers I don't drive much, just to be safe. But then how will all the errands get done? Besides, I compensate pretty well. I'm extremely cautious on the road, and I stick close to home: groceries, small errands, and that sort of thing. I leave the bigger trips to Denny.

Today is one of those bigger trips. We visit my doctor in Lincoln to discuss the possibility of having another child. I haven't had a period since the aneurysm, almost two years, so I'm wondering if it's even possible. The news is disappointing.

"You may not be able to have another child." My doctor explains to us that on the outside, I look like a twenty-six-year-old, but on the inside, I am more like a sixty-year-old. That's why I'm not having a period. The aneurysm had taken a toll on my female organs. I guess I just thought the damage is mainly in my brain. I don't realize how extensively it affects the rest of my body.

We leave his office quietly, giving his words time to sink in. Once in the car, heading home, I turn to Denny and say, "Might not, right?"

"Right."

"That's not no, then."

"No, but you haven't had a period for a long time now, Bec. Besides, if you do get pregnant, it will be much rougher on your body than when we had Aimee."

"But it's what we want, isn't it?"

Denny reaches for my hand. "Yes, but not if it means you could get hurt."

"I don't want to live like that. No fears or what ifs. Let's just leave it in God's hands."

I lay my head back and relax. Denny is quiet for a long time.

Now it's my turn to reassure him. "It'll be okay. I know it."

He kisses my hand. "Okay."

I can feel his lips trembling.

THREE MONTHS LATER

BECKI

I almost gave up hope of ever having a period again. I hadn't had a period since my aneurysm. Listen to me! What woman in her right mind would say such a thing? I used to think periods were a curse from God because Eve had to pick that stinkin' apple. But now, it'd be a blessing, and I'd savor every cramp. And just when I was about to forget the whole thing, God surprises me.

"Denny!" I yell and run out of the bathroom.

"What's the matter?" He rushes to me. "Your head okay?"

"No, that's not it." I scoop Aimee up along with her stuffed animal and swing them both in the air. "You just need to go to the store. I don't have any pads."

Denny stares at me for a moment. "Are you kidding?"

"Nope." I giggle and hug Aimee. "It's official. I have my period."

"All right." Denny hugs us both, but the ever-cautious scientist adds, "But don't get your hopes up too much."

I roll my eyes at him. "I know. I know!"

Denny smiles. "Okay, I'll be back in a bit."

After he leaves, the cramps start full force. So, I celebrate each one over a bowl of ice cream with Aimee. And we soon get the OK from my obstetrician to get pregnant again. He thinks my body is healthy enough and might be functioning well enough to get pregnant, but he cautions us not to be overly optimistic.

SIX MONTHS LATER

BECKI

I lost the baby. I wasn't even sure if I was pregnant, but as soon as I started hemorrhaging, I knew.

Denny was sad too, but we're not going to give up. We're going to try again. He takes me to the doctor, and it isn't very encouraging. I hoped I could stop taking the Dilantin and phenobarbital; maybe they were what caused the miscarriage. But the doctor thinks that's a bad idea. I need the drugs to stop any future seizures.

Denny and I know the risks. Our child could be born with a disability. But we look at it like this: when Aimee was conceived, we knew we'd love her regardless of any imperfections. When our second child is born, we'll love him or her too, no matter what.

FINALLY – A SPEECH THERAPIST

BECKI

We finally find a speech therapist in Norfolk to help me with my language and comprehension skills. We meet just once a week and before long, I find out we may be leaving Norfolk. But it is a start, and I think she has helped me quite a bit.

CHAPTER 6

The Journey Continues
Another New Place

SPRING 1979, WE'RE MOVING

Becki

DENNY HAS THE OPPORTUNITY TO move to the main office of the Nebraska Geological Survey at the University of Nebraska campus in Lincoln. Although our time in Norfolk has been a very important growing experience for us, and the people we have met here are just fantastic, this is a good opportunity for Denny. He started the first one-person office for the geological survey in Norfolk, now he will be able to get more involved with other activities at the University in Lincoln.

We start getting ready to sell our house. But before we begin moving too fast with things, Denny ships Aimee and me back to my parents in Elgin for about a month so he can finally finish his thesis and receive his master's degree from University of Wisconsin-Milwaukee. He has been trying to finish and submit his final draft ever since we moved into our house. He set up a table in the basement and laid everything out on it. However, his progress was the epitome of "two steps forward and one step backward." He would have spurts of time when he would make good progress, but then it would sit for too long while he was attending to his full-time job and to his husband and father duties, especially given the extra time he spent helping me gain back my life.

Sometimes he would only make up the one step backward he had lost before the thesis would lay idle again. But now he is running out of time to complete it without filing for an extension. He takes a couple weeks of vacation from work while we are in Elgin and focuses on completing his final draft, then submitting it, and defending it. His advisor gives him the sage advice: "Don't worry about it being perfect; it will already be wrong the day after you defend it. Just get it done!"

In late March, Denny goes straight to Milwaukee from Norfolk for his thesis defense. Then he picks Aimee and me up in Elgin and we head back to Norfolk. It is a great relief for him to be done and it allows him to focus on the move to Lincoln and attend to his family full-time again.

MEETING OUR WATERLOO

BECKI

This weekend Denny and I are going with Aimee back to Wisconsin for Denny's brother's high school graduation. We are driving across northern Iowa and Denny is getting sleepy so he asks me if I can drive. I have had my license back for about two years now and have been driving quite a bit again. Since there isn't too much traffic (after all—it is northern Iowa), I am feeling pretty confident about driving again since my last seizure was more than two years ago. One thing I do need to watch out for though is farm tractors.

As I am driving down the highway, I come up behind one of those slow green monsters. I think, *No problem, I'll just zip right around it.* But as I start to pass the tractor, I suddenly feel a boom .

I think the loss of peripheral vision in my right eye alters my judgment of the speed of the tractor, and I clip the back left tire of the tractor as I try to pass it. Then, to make matters worse, those huge tires pick up the front end of our 1968 Chevy Nova and fling us to the side, then into the ditch and up against a barbed wire fence..

We are banged up, but no serious injuries other than Denny's broken nose, facial scratches, and my sore back. Thank God Aimee is OK!

The local rescue team from the city of Allison, Iowa, takes us to the hospital in Waterloo, where we are quickly patched up. The wife of one of the paramedics even takes Aimee to her home and watches her while Denny and I go to the hospital. They are really wonderful, caring people (after all – it is Iowa!).

Although we are a bit shaken up, we keep going. We rent a car in Waterloo and forge ahead. We always remember this trip as "meeting our Waterloo in Waterloo." And our poor '68 Nova finds its eternal resting place in a junkyard in Allison, Iowa.

MOVE TO LINCOLN

BECKI

We move again, (of course during the hottest week of July). Denny will work in the main office of the geological survey at the University of Nebraska, in Lincoln. Go Big Red!

Because we looked for houses in Lincoln for a while and couldn't find one, when our house in Norfolk suddenly sold, Denny ended up making an offer on a house in Lincoln without my even seeing it. I'm not sure how many wives would let this happen. Less than 1,000 square feet, it is a well-built two-bedroom home and perfect for us. We buy it from the original owners, who had it custom-built.

The house is close to the university and to Madonna Rehabilitation Hospital, a specialized rehabilitation hospital for stroke patients and other people with a traumatic brain injury. My neurologist gave us the name of a highly recommended speech pathologist at Madonna. Now Denny can spend more time at home instead of traveling back and forth between Lincoln and Norfolk, and I have access to a speech pathologist. I can finally start therapy again.

The Journey Continues—Another New Place

FALL 1979—PNEUMONIA ALMOST GOT ME

BECKI

Denny comes home from work and I am lying on the couch hardly able to talk or move. Fortunately, Aimee is keeping herself occupied playing with her "little people"—thank heavens for Fischer Price. Although I have been through a lot in the last several years, I can't remember feeling as badly as I feel now. I have no energy and have an awful pain in my chest. Denny doesn't think I look good so he takes me to the emergency room.

Before I can protest, I am lying in a hospital bed again, this time with pneumonia. We know that my resistance is probably not what it should be due to my stroke and, in particular, the lung problems I had shortly after surgery. But I'm not ready for this.

My mom comes to help Denny with Aimee and me. She seems concerned with the way things are going. When my mom, the nurse, is concerned, then I'm concerned too. She keeps checking my temperature to see if the fever is breaking. She brings me water. I know that look on her face because I saw it many times when I was in the hospital four years ago.

The length of my stay without improvement has my mom even more worried. But thankfully, after about two weeks, the doctors finally discover that I have a rather rare strain of bacteria causing the pneumonia and they are able to finally find the right antibiotic.

This was somewhat of a scare though, having survived a severe hemorrhagic stroke and then almost getting zapped by a little-known bug. I guess the Lord still has a plan for me to stick around for a while longer. I have to tease Mom a little though.

"Gee, Mom," I say. "Didn't we just go through this about four years ago?"

WINTER 1979 TO 1980—THE MEETING

BECKI

Butterflies are not just fluttering, they are popping out of my stomach as I walk into Madonna for my first session with my new speech therapist, Julie. I keep thinking, *What if this doesn't work? What if I'm a lost cause? Will I be sentenced to a lifetime of struggling with my words, having to pause while I dig through my brain to push out words?*

Never mind. I blink the thoughts away and approach the receptionist.

"May I help you?" She smiles and waits for me as I gather my thoughts.

"Here for therapy with Julie."

She nods and runs her finger through the appointment book in front of her. "Oh, yes, Becki. I think you'll like her." Then she directs her attention to Aimee and her handful of books to keep her occupied.

"Why don't you let us entertain your daughter while you go for your therapy session?"

I think she can see distrust written on my face.

"I promise we'll take good care of her," she laughs. "No straightjackets or padded rooms."

I can feel my jitters disappearing.

"Here, let me show you." She motions us to follow her and leads us to a small room with five adults who were probably in their fifties.

"This is where some of our stroke patients come to relax while they wait for their appointments. I'm sure they would love to read with your daughter."

I'm still not convinced.

"My name's Jan." She points to a nurse talking with a resident. "That's Sister Margie and she can get things rolling."

Sister Margie walks over and shakes my hand. After the introductions are taken care of, Sister Margie bends down to talk to Aimee. "How would you like us to read those books to you?"

Aimee looks up at me for reassurance. I nod, "It's okay, Aimee. Go ahead, Mommy will be back after you're done reading." Aimee hesitates for a moment and then hands Sister Margie a book.

"Oh, this is a good one," Sister Margie says and sits down with Aimee.

I follow Jan to the speech pathologist's office, and look back one last time. Aimee is sitting next to Sister Margie absorbed in her book. One of the patients has joined them.

THE READING TEST

BECKI

The meeting starts out wonderfully. We talk about our families, move on to my new house, my parents, and dive right into my aneurysm and recovery.

Then Julie, my well-dressed speech pathologist, gives me a test.

She makes me read the paragraph. At first, I try to distract her and get her thinking about something else. But she is focused on that damned piece of paper in front of her with the lines and words. Words I know I won't be able to read very well and probably won't comprehend when I am done.

I don't know if it's better to live in denial or face it. I'll flunk.

"I can't read," I sigh.

She smiles and says amicably, "You're whining."

"But my reading is terrible."

She leans forward and looks me squarely in the face. "You don't have to hide it from me. I'm going to help you."

So, I read the damned paragraph and only recognize and understand two of the words in the first sentence. I shake my head. I believe she wants to help me, but I feel so frustrated. Aimee can read better than I can.

"We've got time. Don't worry about that. Just take your time."

I try again. I have no clue if I'm reading the words correctly or not. It's humiliating and excruciatingly slow. I can't say half the words, much less understand them. When I'm finished, I look at Julie.

She says, "OK, Becki, can you tell me in your own words what was said in the paragraph."

I try not to, but I start crying because I have no idea. "I don't know what I just read. Here I am taking care of my daughter, and I can't even read a paragraph."

"No, no. It's a different process. The aneurysm affected the part of your brain that deals with how you process words. But you are smart," she assures me. "You've lost the ability to read like you once did, but you can relearn that. And I can see that you've regained so much already just by what you've told me; that takes a lot of cleverness and ingenuity." She hands me a tissue.

I blow my nose and take a deep breath. I nod at her. "Okay."

"Okay," she says.

We start again.

AIMEE THE ENCOURAGER

BECKI

"And the gi-n-g-er b-bread man ran fast-er and faster." Aimee points to each word as I say it.

"That's good, Mommy!" She smiles at me. "Keep going!"

Aimee keeps her finger under each word so I won't get lost as I finish reading the last few pages of *The Gingerbread Man* to her. It's exhausting, but I keep going because it's such a joy to finally be able to read to her. I still get stuck on words, but my little teacher is helping me along. She and I are learning to sound out the words together.

Speech therapy is helping me. While Aimee is reading books with Sister Margie and the day patients at Madonna, I am relearning how to form my words and read with Julie. I guess I'm not a lost cause after all.

FEBRUARY 1980—OUR MIRACLE

BECKI

God does work in mysterious ways. I'm pregnant again!

My obstetrician in Lincoln, who we started with when we first moved to Norfolk, is close to retirement, so he refers me to a new obstetrician, who is experienced with high-risk pregnancies. This time, the doctor will monitor my progress monthly. He checks my blood pressure, vital signs, and feels my stomach. Then, before I leave, he gives me that serious look and says, "Make sure you keep taking your meds."

I just smile at him and nod. I won't forget. A mixture of joy and overwhelming awe fills my heart. God continues to bless me, and I won't take it for granted. Thank you, I whisper, knowing that He's listening, sure that He's always been listening.

SUMMER 1980—GRADUATION

BECKI

"Bec, I think this is graduation," Julie says to me out of the blue.

"Huh?" I can't believe what she's saying.

"Keep busy." She continues not even noticing the dazed look on my face. "Stop by Madonna whenever you want."

"But I'm not ready!"

"Yes, you are. I've done all I can. Your word retrieval has improved greatly and your speech is much more fluid. Now, the rest is up to you."

112

"What do I have to do?"

"Just keep talking." She leans against her desk and winks at me. "You're good at that."

I look down at my expanding belly. "Well, I guess this is it, Little One. Your mommy is officially graduated and repaired." Then I look up at Julie.

"Thank you. I don't know what I would have done without your help."

Julie smiles at me. "Knowing you, Becki, you would still have done a lot."

NOVEMBER 1980—ABIE ARRIVES

BECKI

"Don't push, Becki!" says Dr. Hanson.

"MMmf, got to."

"Listen to the doctor, hon," Denny tells me.

Listen to the doctor? He's not even my doctor. He's just filling in for him. Where was Dr. Bakus, anyway? I'm getting worried here. Does this guy know what he's doing?

The need is so strong, but if I push too hard, I'm afraid I could rupture the veins in my head or go into a grand mal seizure, putting me and my baby at risk. I don't feel any headaches right now, so that's a good sign, isn't it? Please Lord, get me through this.

"You're doing great, Bec." Denny's standing next to the doctor watching my progress like a football game going into overtime. "Come on, Bec, you can do it!"

I concentrate hard on NOT pushing when a swoosh of water splashes to the floor. My water breaks, and soon I hear a baby's cry as it's pulled into the world.

The doctor shakes his head. "You did it, Becki, without any pushing. Wait until Dr. Bakus hears this one!"

Denny brings her to me, beaming from ear to ear. "We have another beautiful baby girl."

I begin to cry. "Abie," I whisper. "Our little miracle."

DENNY

After Becki delivers Abie, I overhear Dr. Hanson telling the medical student who was observing the delivery that he may never again witness a delivery without any pushing.

Abie was delivered during a normal contraction. I guess those many weeks we spent in Lamaze class, learning the breathing techniques, paid off. And the Dilantin and phenobarbital she takes to slow down her brain and nervous system activity probably helped also.

Less than a week after Becki delivers Abie, it's my turn to go to the hospital—for hemorrhoid surgery. Becki's mom is coming out to help us with our new addition, so we thought it was a good time for me to get that taken care of. It seems a little odd that Becki delivers the baby and I have hemorrhoid surgery. You should have seen us fighting over the donut pillow.

JULY 1981—A SURPRISE VISITOR

BECKI

Out of the blue I get the call from Julie, my speech pathologist, asking me to visit Madonna. She entices me with the words, "We have a speaker coming next week. You might be interested in her."

I might, but it has to be pretty good. With two little ones to care for, I'm becoming choosy on which things I will leave them for, even if it is only for a few hours. "Who is it?" I ask.

"Patricia Neal."

There's a pause as I try to absorb what she just said.

"Do you know who that is?" Julie asks.

Give me a break! I have brain damage, but I'm not stupid. Of course, I know who she is. She's only one of the best actresses there is! I must've seen *The Miracle Worker* a dozen times I can't believe it. "Of course, I do!"

"Well, good, because she's coming here next week to speak to the stroke patients. "And," she emphasizes this part, "Patricia Neal wants to meet you."

"Excuse me?!"

"She wants to meet some of the stroke patients," Julie explains, "and since her stroke is very similar to yours, I told her about you. I hope you don't mind. Now she wants to meet you. It's on a Sunday and I thought you, Denny, and the girls could come to my office. I really hope you can make it."

Julie waits for me to respond. When I don't, she asks again, "Well, will you?"

In my excitement, I start pacing the floor, accidentally wrapping the telephone cord around myself. "Of course," I tell her as I twirl backward to untangle myself. All the while, Aimee is giggling like I'm the best show in town. Abie catches her sister's enthusiasm and starts to bounce up and down in her jumpy seat. Pretty soon, we're all laughing.

STARSTRUCK

BECKI

After church, Denny and I take the girls to Madonna to meet Ms. Neal. Aimee, in the hopes that one of the patients will read to her like they did in the past, brings a stack of books. "That's okay," I think because it will keep her and Abie somewhat occupied until Sister Margie brings Ms. Neal to the office.

We must look like such a sight. Denny looks pretty calm, but I know otherwise. His knuckles are white from squeezing the armrest so tightly. Me, on the other hand, I try to keep my brain focused on the children. I stand and rock Abie, and rehearse our meeting in my head. If she says, "Hello." What do I say? "Hello, Ms. Neal. Hello, Patricia." *Do I curtsey like you do for royalty?* She is a big movie star, you know. *Oh, God, I just hope I don't make a fool of myself.*

Soon the door opens and I can feel my stomach drop. It's her. She looks radiant, and I wonder if all stars have that glow. Then I wonder how she could've had a stroke. She doesn't look like she could even break a nail.

Sister Margie begins the pleasantries. I swallow hard when she introduces me. *Okay,* I tell myself, *just open your mouth when it's time and say hello.*

Sister Margie motions to me. "And this is Becki."

116

Ms. Neal steps closer and points at me and in her deep voice says, "I want to talk to you."

Denny elbows me, and I know just what he's thinking because I'm thinking the same thing. *I'm in for it now.*

"You are Rebecca, correct?"

I nod. I feel like a naughty child about to be scolded.

"Sister Margie and your speech therapist told me that you've had a very severe stroke." Ms. Neal has a talent for emphasizing every word. "What you must do now, is never, NEVER stop fighting. And if you never stop fighting, you will always be the winner."

After that, she goes back to the lobby to mingle with everyone else before her presentation. I listen to her story and think to myself, this woman is a warrior — a glamorous warrior! She never let her stroke defeat her. She's definitely a lady in charge of her life.

Before she leaves, she pulls me aside one more time. Lowering her eyes at me, she says, "Don't forget."

"I won't," I promise, feeling empowered by her example. "Thank you."

From now on, I will be a warrior, too.

1981 TO 1985—LIFE GOES ON

BECKI

Over the next several years, life starts to become a little bit more routine, even though I still have my ongoing reading and comprehension challenges, I am becoming a master of adaptation and compensation.

I now have two small children to care for. Aimee starts grade school so we become very involved in our Lutheran school. We are involved in parent-teacher league and Denny is on the school board.

I start selling Avon and babysitting for some friends from our church to help our income. Denny and I become counselors for the senior high youth group at our church, we assist with spaghetti dinners and musicals, and interact with many wonderful youths. We even attend Narcotics Anonymous meetings to help out one young lady who has some significant challenges.

One of the things Denny continues to do to help me recover my motor skills is to play tennis with me. Well—we may not really be "playing" tennis, but rather we try to see if I can move beyond hitting the ball into the net every time. We go to the tennis courts just a couple blocks from our house. We take Aimee and Abie with us and "coax" them into being ball retrievers for us, which given my situation keeps them extremely busy. There is a Dairy Queen across the street so we bribe them with Dilly Bars. Some people may consider this to be child abuse, but the promise of a chocolate or cherry Dilly Bar keeps the girls from reporting us to the local authorities.

SPRING 1986—BEING PUBLISHED

BECKI

I am writing a book with the help of a student from our church youth group. Her name is Linda. She's interested in becoming a speech pathologist, and after I suggest it, she starts volunteering at Madonna to get some experience. Now I guess I'm her experiment. She visits me a couple times a week and guides me through the process of writing. She says, "Writing will help you become a better reader." Sometimes I think it's helping, but other times, it's just plain overwhelming.

I'm writing, in my own words, the Biblical story about the Jews being held as slaves. God sends Moses to free them and brings them to the Promised Land. I put the title in big letters, "LET MY PEOPLE GO."

Writing the story is taking forever, but it is giving me hope. If God can free thousands of slaves and part the sea for their escape to a new life, then healing me should be a snap. Linda's sister, who is an artist, does fantastic illustrations for the book.

I dedicate the book to Dr. Uttech, the neurosurgeon who spent several hours helping me regain my life on the late evening on that fateful day back on February 1, 1976. We have a friend who is an attorney, and he helps me get a copyright for my book. I am now "published"!

Because Linda is taking speech pathology classes at the university, I offer to make presentations to several classes about my experience as a stroke survivor with aphasia. I really do enjoy speaking to people about my experience, hopefully helping the future speech pathologists understand how the brain of an aphasic works, or sometimes doesn't work.

CHAPTER 7

ON THE MOVE AGAIN
BACK TO WISCONSIN

FALL 1986—A QUAINT LITTLE TOWN AND
ANOTHER UNPRODUCTIVE DOCTOR APPOINTMENT

BECKI

Denny has always had good luck when it comes to choosing a home for us. Denny took a new job with an environmental consulting firm in Milwaukee, Wisconsin, and said he found a townhouse for us to temporarily rent in a quaint little town called Cedarburg. My trust in his taste is unquestionable (he picked me, right?), so in November, 1986, we packed up our belongings and moved to Cedarburg, about 15 miles north of Milwaukee. We initially move into the townhouse, then eventually into a cozy ranch-style home.

This, hopefully, will be our last move. As the girls get older, we want to be able to raise them in one community. Every day, as I learn more and more about this town, I know we made the right decision. The neighbors are friendly, bringing us treats and introducing themselves. There are young children here, too, so Aimee, who is in 6th grade, will soon have babysitting jobs and Abie, who is in kindergarten, will have playmates.

I have to say, Denny's first description of the town was also right on the money when he said it was like something out of a Currier and Ives Christmas painting. It is quaint with its historical buildings lining the main street. Everyone seems to know everyone, too. Sometimes I wonder if we haven't actually stepped onto the set of *The Andy Griffith Show* (minus the town drunk) instead of downtown Cedarburg.

DENNY

Once we get settled in our townhouse, I make an appointment with a neurologist in Milwaukee for Becki. Dr. Becker passed away and Dr. Uttech no longer practices. Anyway, they were neurosurgeons and now we should have a neurologist for Becki. But I certainly was not expecting our appointment to go the way it did.

I understand the doctor has to ask a lot of questions, but he seems particularly impatient with the clarity and timeliness of Becki's answers. I thought, "Why do you think we are here in the first place? She has aphasia."

Becki was very upset about the encounter. I guess we learn that even many medical professionals don't understand how the brain of a person with aphasia works—that communication and comprehension are their biggest challenges.

On the Move Again—Back to Wisconsin

BECKI

Once Aimee and Abie are both in school, I decide it is time to try to join the workforce. At first, I try a job at a local fast-food restaurant. Denny helps me fill out the application, but it is just too fast-paced and stressful. I can't process what people are directing me to do as fast as they are doing it. After that fiasco, I decide to contact the local vocational rehabilitation office to help me find a job better suited to my abilities.

The vocational rehabilitation office helps people with disabilities find and keep jobs in the community. That's what I need. After all these years of not working, and with my difficulty reading and comprehending, I have to admit, I need help.

First, I undergo some psychological testing that I would like to erase. My reading abilities are assessed at a 4th-grade level and my comprehension at a 3.8-grade level. As a former English major, having to hear this is painful enough without also hearing one person's assessment. The Ph.D. psychologist, who seems to be devoid of any personality, suggests that I have unreasonable employment expectations due to my lack of communication skills and that I should work in a sheltered setting, participate in a day program (daycare for adults), or file for Social Security Disability Insurance (SSDI).

How dare he assess me like that after just one short visit! He doesn't know how I've struggled; how far I've come. He doesn't know how hard I fought to get to this point. I can hear Ms. Neal's voice in my head. I mean, she has won an Academy Award, a Tony Award, a Golden Globe Award, and two British Academy Film Awards. She knows my successes. *Never give up.* That's when the warrior in me kicks in. How can he make a judgment on

123

me based on a few tests? He can't. I won't let him. I have a goal. Whether he likes it or not, I am going to get a job.

Then I am referred to a sheltered workshop for training, a place that assists people with disabilities to work in either a self-contained setting or supported employment with a job coach. I am hoping for supported employment so that maybe, eventually, I can work without any help at all.

Before I can start any training at the sheltered workshop, I am given a vocational evaluation. To my relief, it is a bit more favorable. Although the results of this test are humbling, it isn't humiliating. According to the results, I have verbal and comprehension problems, with comprehension being the most impaired.

Most of this information I already know. I have difficulty reading and hearing directions and filling out informational forms on the test. I also have to restate what the evaluator says, and that is extremely difficult. In the evaluator's opinion, immediate recall of information is my biggest problem. No kidding!

This evaluator does give me hope, though. Instead of saying I should collect SSDI, she says they can train me for a job in the area of activity aide. I could help recreation and activity therapists in nursing homes, residential centers, or hospitals.

I can work!

THE ACTIVITY AIDE

BECKI

The vocational rehab people found me an opportunity as an activity aide with a local social services agency. My job is to help organize activities for senior citizens who come to a facility as day patients. I guess even though I went through the vocational rehab process and have all the testing and psychological evaluations, it still must be hard for them to really understand and explain to a potential employer what my abilities and disabilities are. I think it is especially difficult for people to understand how the mind and communication of an aphasic works.

My supervisor talks so fast when explaining to me what she wants me to do, that by the time she is done I have only understood about 20 percent of what she said. Needless to say, only being able to follow 20 percent of the instructions for your job doesn't lead to a good working situation. I start to think that maybe that Ph.D. psychologist was right—that I should just apply for SSDI because maybe I'm not employable.

But then that thought makes me even madder and I am bound and determined that I am going to show them (whoever *them* is) that I can work. I decide I am probably going to have to seek out the right opportunity in my own time and on my own conditions.

THE FLOWER SHOP

BECKI

Since I am told I can work, I am pounding the pavement pretty hard. My first few attempts are minor disasters. The fast-food industry was just too fast-paced for me, and the activity aide supervisor's instructions were too fast, although I think I would have been good at that job, with a little patience.

I thought working in a flower shop at a supermarket would be interesting, but when I try to apply at one that is looking for help, I am politely told the position is filled. This is after I am given an application and asked to fill it out. I sit down at a table in the back and try to read the questions, but it is futile.

When one of the managers comes back to check on my progress, he doesn't look too pleased. He picks up the paper and says, "Thank you, we'll let you know if another position opens up." I know what that means, and I am embarrassed and a bit hurt. When I tell him that I have a disability and that it takes me longer to read things than most other people, I can see he changes his tune because he is afraid I might sue him for discrimination. I just nod and get out of there as fast as I can.

Once outside, I put my head on the steering wheel and cry. So many years have passed, and it still stings when others see my disability and dismiss me like I'm not even worth a minute of their time.

Forget it, I tell myself and put the key in the ignition. There'll be something else. I wipe the tears away and drive home.

BACK TO SCHOOL—
SPECIAL EDUCATION PARAPROFESSIONAL

BECKI

I know I want to work with people, so I try the local school districts next. Maybe that will be a more pleasant experience than fast food, activity aide, or flower shops with impatient supervisors.

Finally, my luck changes. I land a job on my own as a special education paraprofessional, in a neighboring school district. I will be working with students at the high school. I am so excited. My first REAL job since that Sunday morning twelve years ago when my life changed forever.

My daughters, on the other hand, are a bit wary. "Who will eat cookies with me after school?" asks Abie.

They don't ask for help with their homework, because I just can't help them much. It is something understood between the girls and me, but disheartening nevertheless. I can, however, help children with intellectual or developmental challenges participate in school activities. I am a pro at modifying my own surroundings to be a successful wife and mother, and I have no doubt I can do the same for children with disabilities.

SATISFIED

BECKI

Well, it's been quite a ride so far. Sometimes it's a bit overwhelming; you never know what will happen next. You're lucky if you get to sit down for two seconds, but working with these students is one of the most rewarding experiences of my life.

When a student looks up at me, just waiting for me to help him understand something, I can see the struggle in his face, and I can feel it as if it is my own. When I help a child succeed, it's as if I have succeeded too. When a student is finally able to tie her shoelaces after the 100th time trying, or count to 20 without skipping a number, or read ½ on the measuring cup so she can finish her cooking assignment, I know I'm making a difference.

A SPECIAL SWIMMER

BECKI

I may never step into a pool again.

I have been assigned to one of our larger students. He can be quite stubborn to the point of becoming physical if we push him too hard. I should've remembered that before I entered the pool with him during gym class. But in my defense, Joe usually loves the water.

Everything is okay during warm-up activities. We stretch our arms, jump up and down, and twist left and right. Joe watches me and follows, but keeps a safe distance from me. Things change, though, when we have to swim to the deeper part. My life flashes before my eyes when Joe decides he doesn't like the deep water anymore.

Of course, I have to try and get him to do a few strokes out there. He can swim and our goal is to have him build up his muscle strength by treading water for a few minutes. Joe has a different plan. He decides to use me as a chair and sit like a king in the deeper water. He pushes me down and tries to get on top of me. I struggle to remove his hand from my neck and start thrashing around. Dammit! Where are the other teachers and lifeguard? I feel like I am under forever.

Somehow, I manage to wiggle out of his grasp and sneak behind him. He can't figure out where I am until I come back up beside him. He still looks angry and is about to push me under when I place my hand on the top of his head and push him down for a second instead. Joe comes up and stares at me in disbelief.

Still trying to catch my breath, I say, "Joe, don't you EVER do that to me again! You hurt Lawton." I have to make him understand that what he did to me was scary and the only way I can is to make him feel it for a second.

I think both Joe and I learn a big lesson today. Joe learns to respect me, and I learn to do my hair after swim class.

CHAPTER 8
HER LANGUAGE OF LOVE

1988 TO 1995, LIFE BECOMES SOMEWHAT ROUTINE

BECKI

As I now have a job and am using some of the skills I learned in college and in life, our lives just seem to move on somewhat normally, although I still struggle with my speech and language and with my reading.

Aimee graduates from high school in 1993 and heads to Valparaiso University, where Denny and I met and fell in love.

I love knowing I can make a difference in someone's life, even with a disability. But I become more personally aware of my impact on others when Aimee shares this paper she wrote in her college English class.

Her Language of Love (1994)

I paged through each book, reading the backs of every one. "I don't know. I want all of them," I said of the various novels by D. H. Lawrence, Toni Morrison, and other favorites. So far the longest stop on our recent mall trip had been at Waldenbooks. I looked up and was startled by the look on my mother's face. Her eyes were filled with tears. She could barely speak.

131

Hernzebekana! Her Language of Love

"I wish ...," she hesitated to regain her composure. "You may have as many as you want. Don't worry about the price. I'll help you." I knew what was wrong but I didn't press it further. My sister took care of that.

"Mo—om, what's wrong? Did I do something? We're in a bookstore, Mom, stop it." My disapproving glance Abie's way stifled her whining line of questioning. Mom provided the answers in her own time.

Eighteen years earlier, my mother had just been released from the hospital. On February 1, 1976, in a matter of seconds, all the aspirations of the twenty-four-year-old new mother with a college degree were destroyed. There would be no Law School for this English major. A blood clot burst and caused a grand mal seizure on that bitter cold Sunday morning. From that point on, her and her families' life would be changed forever. The complicated brain surgery was successful, but she remained in a coma for several weeks afterwards. God had miraculously spared this young woman's life in a potentially fatal situation. His purpose was unknown at the time.

After a month of fighting her deep sleep, Becki awoke to face the results of her brain damage. The impairments were devastating. She was paralyzed on her right side and blind in half of her right eye. Even worse, this young woman who spent the last six years of her life studying literature, writing, and preparing for law school, had lost her ability to communicate. She couldn't speak, read or write. While her brain was capable of understanding the verbal and written messages around her, she was unable herself to communicate her thoughts and express the words that she could see before her.

Her Language of Love

Therapy began as soon as possible. Physical therapy took first priority. Learning to walk at age twenty-four was humiliating, but she persevered and soon was able to transport herself from place to place without the help of a walker. April quickly rolled around and Becki was released from the hospital under the care of her husband and mother. At that point she was still unable to speak coherently. A friend from childhood worked with her twice a week on reading and writing. As for talking, she practiced for one audience the most—me.

I was too young at the time to be a critic. She stumbled over words, but I didn't judge; her words, attention and love were enough for me. It was then that I started my lessons of language.

As I began to grow physically and intellectually, my mother's endeavors to regain her lost communication skills proved to be an opportunity for learning. It started with verbal challenges and victories. At age two, my grandma, my mom and I were in the car returning home from a visit to relatives. To pass the time, Mommy and I practiced our alphabet. When we reached the letter "h" I stopped.

"H—hydrogeologist!" I blurted. Grandma and Mommy laughed. Daddy was a hydrogeologist; I had heard Mommy use the word before. From that point on I was fed with complex words to add to my limited two-year old vocabulary. It was like introducing fine chocolate to someone who had never tasted anything but cabbage water and potatoes. I was fascinated by "pollution," and

when sunbathing with Mommy, I made sure I "concentrated." As my verbal skills increased I became more and more a critic of my mother.

"No, Mommy. Say it with me, 'mag-a-zine'."

"Mag-a-zine," she complied, and soon I assumed the role of teacher that originally belonged to my mother.

The next stop on my journey of language acquisition was reading and writing. Again, my mother's handicap pushed me along. Up until age four, she could get away with reading stories based on what she saw in the illustrations. They were familiar stories: Three Little Pigs, Goldilocks and the Three Bears, and others. Soon the words began to have meaning for me, and I forced my student to truly read what was on the page.

"That's not what it says, Mommy. You skipped the last sentence before the wolf huffs and puffs?" I caught her.

"Alright," she laughed. "The wolf was fr-fur-fre..."

"Furious, Mommy," I explained. From that point on, she was forced into mastering every children's book on my shelf.

Trips to the library became more frequent and Mommy's new speech pathologist (yet another word to add to my increasing vocabulary) assigned her to read to me every night. Daddy would sit with us too and help Mommy and I with the big words. It wasn't long before Mommy's reading skills surpassed mine. It was easier for her to merely recollect what skills she had lost than it was for me to absorb the new knowledge. My teaching career with my mother was put on hold.

In the meantime, I acquired a new student, my new little sister Abie. Mommy was a much better student than Abie. I couldn't understand why, at age two, she refused to read the words I wrote on the chalkboard: "cat", "hat", "sit". I persisted and once she learned to talk and read, I began to regret my efforts.

High school quickly arrived and soon I surpassed my mother's language skills. Once again I assumed my role as teacher, though with increased patience, for she was becoming more sensitive to her verbal limits. I urged her to practice reading more complex books and even dug out her old novels from the basement, but she declined. "It takes too long, Aimee, you know that", she would argue, but her excuses didn't satisfy me. I could tell that she was embarrassed by her inability to read as quickly as I could. It was a tool that proved useful. As my vocabulary increased, her pride forced hers to increase as well. As she stumbled over new words, I was there to help her along.

"pro—"
"pro-," she repeated.
"cras-"
"cras-"
"tin-"
"ni...ti...tin-, she stumbled.
"ate."
" 'ate."

135

Hernzebekana! Her Language of Love

"p-pro-procrastinate!" she sputtered.

Through it all she was able to laugh. I was never a critic, but I wouldn't let her use her impairment as an excuse. Sometimes she would try to use an easier word, but I forced the original out of her. I knew how important it was for her to understand, to read, and to communicate easily on her own. Soon I didn't have to force her to make the effort. She would come to me for help or work through her struggles alone.

When college approached, it seemed natural for me to major in English. All my life, Mother showed me how important words were. Until the ability to communicate was robbed from her, she took it for granted. She taught me never to do the same. From the very beginning I respected how powerful language is, and understood how vital it was to my mother's survival.

That day in Waldenbooks was a turning point for both of us. The old dusty novels from the basement have finally found their way back into the right hands, hers. On that day I was struck with the realization of what my mother had done for me. I realized to whom I owed my love for words. It was my mother, who through her survival and victories, taught me the most important thing I will ever learn—respect for language, her "language of love."

Her Language of Love

BECKI

Although it takes me a while to read Aimee's paper, I do finish it. It is so hard for me to read that much text. I realize that through all the years of me feeling inadequate with my disability, the Lord has used my disability and struggles to be a model and inspiration not just for my students, but also for my daughter.

This becomes even more so apparent when Aimee sends us a letter she wrote on a train traveling from Germany to France during her junior year overseas.

As she explains while contemplating her future life, I find that my misfortune, disability, and struggles have made an impact that changed Aimee's career path, as she explains in the following passages to Denny and to me:

More Words from Aimee (1995)

Dad—I've made some decisions and I felt I should share them with you first. It seems here as if I exist beyond time—like the world can't possibly be moving forward while I am in Europe. Being here has already given me a sense of independence that I didn't have. You would be proud I think. But it also taught me that there are certain things that one cannot plan for. It's OK to have goals, but to plan your path for achieving it isn't always a good idea. It's hard to handle obstacles without flexibility. Take this trip. I've always wanted to study in Europe, but you could never have convinced me that I should be in Germany. It's strange how things work sometimes. At any rate, you know that I haven't really been sure exactly what I really wanted to do. Recently, I haven't been sure I want to teach. Well, the other day we had a 3 1/2-hour bus trip to Berlin – enough time for me to lose attention and to start examining my life, goals, etc. I've been interested in Speech Pathology for a while now, but have been reluctant to purse it for a number of reasons. Well, I think that I really want to do this now. My ultimate goal is to work with adult trauma victims with aphasia and open an office out of my own home...

Mom—Well, Mom, I'm sure by now if you haven't read Dad's part at least you've interrogated him to find out what I said. Yes, you have to say this word (e.g., interrogated) and look it up if you need to. Don't ask Abie or Dad to help you, wimp. There's a dictionary in my room. Now, I have an assignment for you while I'm gone. I know you're a working woman now, but you have 3 months and 13 days to complete this. Find a book. Any book. One from your collection or from my boxes downstairs. Find a book you like and read it. I know you say it takes too long and you won't get anything out of it. That's why I'm giving you this assignment. Take your time and read a little each time. Get a blank notebook, and each time you read a section, summarize what you just read in the notebook. Then when you continue reading from the book, begin by reading your summary from the last time and then continue. Write as much as you need to and be as specific as possible. When I get back, I expect to find a notebook full of summary from a book. This is not an option. If I can figure out how to travel around Europe by myself, then you can read a book. No "buts"...

Aimee challenged me. I did try to meet her challenge but it didn't work out very well for me. I guess reading comprehension is going to continue to be a problem, especially trying to retain a train of thought for multiple paragraphs.

CHAPTER 9

New Opportunity

1995 TO 1998, MY NEW OPPORTUNITY AND SOME NEW EXPERIENCES

BECKI

Okay, let me just get you up to speed. I lost my job at the nearby school district. My position was eliminated when they disbanded the consolidated special education programs in the county. That's what I was told anyway. I'll try to believe it, but part of me wonders if my trying to start a union for paraprofessionals and aides had anything to do with it. Denny calls me Norma Rae! I guess I've become a bit political these days. My sensitivity to being fairly treated in my own life somehow spilled out into my work setting. I guess I've become kind of a zealot. I'll have to watch that in my new position.

Which brings me to the present. After some part-time and substituting positions for a year, I have a new job in my own hometown. In fall 1995, I start working at the high school with students with special needs again, primarily those with emotional challenges. I really do enjoy developing relationships with the teachers and the kids I see around town. And Abie gets the joy of starting her freshman year in high school knowing her mother might be right around the corner at any time. I guess I'd better behave and not embarrass her, which might be kinda tough for me!

The start of 1996 brings on another new experience, planning our first child's wedding. Aimee gets married in August. Even though I have made it a long way in my recovery journey the last 20 years, it is easy to take things for granted. Being able to see my first daughter get married reminds me of the blessings I have received to just still be alive. I guess God wasn't done with me yet.

In order to try to keep up with Denny—and get to see him more often—I get into biking more and more. I even start doing some training rides with him. I always apologize for slowing him down, but he says it's good for him to actually see the scenery of the places he's been riding around for many years. Once he even admits to me he is struggling to just keep up with the pace I am setting, although I'm not sure I really believe him.

In 1997, Denny and I complete a metric century bicycle ride in Marinette, Wisconsin. The ride ends up being 72 miles, rather than 62, after we take a wrong turn on the course—Denny's fault, not mine.

I feel that completing that metric century is almost the pinnacle of my recovery journey physically, even though I still have some weakness on my right side from the 1976 stroke. I also downhill skied a few times, and didn't even break a leg. And I learned how to cross-country ski, which is physically more challenging than letting gravity and speed propel me down a downhill slope.

We also bought rollerblades—and of course, wrist guards. I was actually better at rollerblading than Denny because apparently I had retained the balance I had learned as a child, and balance on skates is not Denny's strong point. Rollerblading also provided us a Thursday date night, when I would drive to downtown

New Opportunity

Milwaukee, pick Denny up from work, go rollerblading on the Lake Michigan waterfront bike trail and then take in the outdoor jazz concert afterwards. I feel like I am doing pretty well physically and I am looking forward to what lies ahead.

At the start of the 1997 school year my co-worker, Deb, and I help start a new program for our students, taking them to a nearby hospital where they learn how to do various jobs around the hospital and get paid for doing it. I really enjoy helping the students with this opportunity, especially since I was in their shoes almost ten years ago during my stint with vocational rehabilitation. We spend the first half of the school day at the school building, then after lunch we go to the hospital. I also enjoy getting to know the people at the hospital and learning how things work in the medical field. Even though I still have some communication challenges myself, I never miss an opportunity to kibitz with people.

In summer 1998, Denny and I celebrate our 25th wedding anniversary with a trip to the Canadian Rockies. We fly into Edmonton then drive to Jasper, south along the Icefields Highway to Banff, and then to Calgary to fly back home. Although there is awesome beauty everywhere we look, two specific experiences resonate with me the most—walking on the Athabasca Glacier and hiking up the Parker Ridge Trail to view the Saskatchewan Glacier down in a valley not viewable from the road.

After getting to the top of the ridge, I am really pooped and sort of mad at Denny because I don't know why he made me do all that tiring switchback hiking. With the loss of my peripheral vision in my right eye, I do not have a full view of the landscape. Denny slowly moves my head about 30 degrees and right there far below in the valley is this beautiful river of ice. Now you may not think a river of ice is a beautiful thing, but if you are married to a hydrogeologist, you sure better! It's times like this that I reflect back on how blessed I really am to have survived that fateful day in February, 1976, and to have the opportunity to experience God's beauty like this.

* * *

Before school starts in fall 1998, I learn I get to break in the new teacher, Dawn, who'll be working with students who have intellectual disabilities. The high school didn't previously have a formal program for these students because there were only three to four kids a few years past. Now, six students are coming up from the middle school—enough to start a program.

Four of the students need one-on-one assistance with their personal needs throughout the school day. Not too hard of a job for me. My previous job was pretty similar. One great thing about this program, though, is that a new apartment-like setting was built into the high school for the students. It has a kitchen, bathroom, and classroom. I can't wait to start the school year!

THE FIRST DAY WITH DAWN 1998

BECKI

Are we in for it?

I meet my colleagues, and I know we'll get along fine—but there's one student, her name is Sable—who is going to give us a run for our money.

She's tiny with a frail body, the mind of a six-year-old, and a personality full of sass.

It happens like this. Dawn, Deb, and I are all sitting around the table getting to know each other and talking about schedules.

Sable, obviously bored by the discussion, decides to get up and walk over to Dawn, who then pulls up a chair and asks Sable to sit down. Sable gives Dawn a look of contempt and wipes a booger right across her face!

Dawn is in shock for a moment before she regains her composure and gives Sable a time-out. Welcome to the new school year.

IT'S GOING OK

BECKI

I'm starting to get used to this new position. Sable has lightened up a bit too. Sometimes she scratches and refuses to do her work, but no boogers have left her nose (which is quite a blessing).

I've become good friends with Deb and Dawn too. We've been dressing up for homecoming week with the kids. Today is Green Bay Packers day. Tomorrow it's pajama day. That's the easy part.

I've also made friends with some of the new students with emotional challenges and reconnected with those I have worked with the past couple of years, some kids other people may be uncomfortable with because they can't look past their exteriors.

Alex is one of those kids. He always wears black, draped with chains, and his face is always painted white. He looks like a bad version of a Kiss band member. To top it all off, he threatens anyone who says hello to him. Well, I do more than say hello. I let him know I can see him behind all that makeup and negativity. I know he just wants some attention, and I give it to him.

Every time I pass Alex in the hall, I say, "Hello." His response is always, "Don't talk to me." Then I say something like, "If I don't talk to you, can I borrow your chains so I can play jump rope with them after school?"

I keep this up every day until finally he cracks a smile. I made a connection. Now, he still says, "Don't talk to me," but it's light-hearted and I've become a safe haven for him. I've let him know he can talk to me anytime.

The people part is the easiest. The hard part is the actual curriculum. I can teach the lifeskill activities like cleaning up the kitchen, doing the laundry, and setting the table. Measuring out things is more difficult, though.

Luckily, Deb takes care of tube-feeding one of our students because it's hard for me to read the tube and make sure to pour the right amount of medicine and Ensure into her tube.

I can help the kids with their math and money problems because they're functioning at a kindergarten to second grade level, which is lower than my abilities. Reading recipes isn't too bad either because Denny and my mom have drilled basic recipes into my head. I am known to make the best macaroni and cheese in my household (according to the experts, my kids). So, I'm successful here because I have a purpose, challenges just like everyone else. Plus, if I have problems, Dawn or Deb are there to help.

It feels like my home away from home, my second family.

CHAPTER 10

BOOM AGAIN!

OCTOBER 1998

DENNY

I haven't said too much lately because this is Becki's story. When her story began, she couldn't speak for herself so I was her voice. She can speak now. I sometimes watch her in amazement at how far she's come. I look at our girls who are closer to being women, and I see their mother's strength and beauty in their faces. Becki taught them how to be strong; how to be fighters, and how to enjoy every day of their lives.

And I feel blessed that I can sit across from Bec at the dinner table and talk about all the things that happen during the day; that we even have a day to share, and I pray that there will be more to come. Every ordinary day is extraordinary because when we wake up, it's a gift from God.

NO! NOT AGAIN!
(from Chapter 1, p. 8—10, Flash Forward)

BECKI

When we go to bed Sunday night, Denny says, "It's been a good weekend," and it truly was.

147

Hernzebekana! Her Language of Love

I feel blessed to be working in the high school special education program, blessed by my family, and proud of my two beautiful daughters, Aimee and Abie. Everything in my world seems perfect. I cuddle up next to Denny and close my eyes.

As I'm just starting to fall asleep, a stabbing pain runs through the back of my head. "Ooh," I groan and jerk backward.

Denny rolls over and faces me. "You okay?"

"Yeah," I say, and I'm not lying, because the pain disappears as quickly as it comes. "Just a little twinge."

In a few hours though, the pain is back and unrelenting. It feels like someone's probing inside my brain. Denny gives me Tylenol, but it doesn't ease the pain. If anything, it's worse. Maybe if I reposition myself, it'll stop. I roll over onto my stomach and cover the back of my head with both hands, trying to stop the threat creeping through my brain. Then I feel something shift, and I panic.

The invisible monster is back.

The pressure continues to build on the left side of my head. It's like déjà vu, and although now I'm forty-six, I feel like that twenty-four-year-old woman again, lying in my bed wondering when this headache will end. This time though, I'm not only wondering when it will end, but how.

I can't go through this again.

Now, once again the steady pounding inside my head shatters the quiet of an early morning, and I cling to the reassurance of Denny's rhythmic soft breaths against my cheek. Abie is sleeping like a baby, although now a young lady, a senior in high school.

Boom Again!

"Denny," I say and nudge him slightly. "Can you get me some water?"

He nods sleepily and refills the water glass next to me.

Please God, I beg, not again. I make up all kinds of excuses. I have a new job. I'm too old to go through this again. We're finally taking that romantic trip to San Francisco we'd dreamed about. Abie still needs me at home, and so on.

Still the pounding continues. I can't believe, after twenty-two years, it is happening again.

Then the realization that this isn't going to go away sinks in. I call out to Denny, barely audible, choking on each word. "Denny, I'm doing it again," like I have any control over it. I know I have none.

I hear the glass in Denny's hand shatter to the bathroom floor and realize I won't be going to work today.

I know I have to be brave. There must be another blood vessel breaking open somewhere inside my head, just like before. I bury my face in the pillow and close my eyes tightly, trying to keep myself together, trying to stay in control. I know I have to muster the courage to go through this again.

DENNY

Becki's eyes are puffy and I can't even imagine the pain she's in, but she's still conscious. I get her into the car and yell to Abie as she runs out to see what's going on. "I have to take Mom to the hospital. Go to school, and I'll call you later."

I can see fear draining the color from Abie's face. She knows what could happen when her mom gets a headache. Becki takes her hand from her head for a second and reaches for Abie. "It'll be okay, Ab. Go to school."

"I'll get a message to school as soon as I can," I tell her and drive off feeling guilty for leaving Abie like that and scared for Becki and myself. Would I lose Becki this time?

I call ahead to let them know we are coming, so as soon as we go through the emergency doors, Becki is taken in for a CAT scan. They find small leaks around the site of her last AVM and need to get her to the hospital in Milwaukee to have a neurosurgeon check things out. It looks like Becki may have to have brain surgery again.

BECKI

Oh, God, I'm so scared. I don't think I can do this again. At least the first time I didn't know what hit me.

This time I know.

They're going to shave my head, open up my skull and close the blood vessels. When I wake up, I'll be trapped inside my head again. I'll be unable to share my thoughts, control my arms and legs—a prisoner in my own body.

"You have to do this," Denny keeps telling me. "You have no choice."

"No, no. I can't," I cry. How can he understand what it's like? This isn't supposed to happen again. People don't live through these things twice.

"Becki, you're going to come out of it better than last time. You may have to go through some rehabilitation again, but I'll help you. You're not going to be alone."

Denny. Always the voice of reason. His words are soothing, and I try to believe him. "Okay." I squeeze his hand wondering if it will be the last time I'll feel his touch. "But don't leave me."

"Never." He says with so much determination, I almost believe he can make it all better.

DENNY

Becki's parents, Cal and Velda, arrive in Milwaukee, mid-afternoon. By then, the neurosurgeon is able to evaluate Becki further. He lays out a couple options for treatment but says he thinks the best approach is to perform surgery to remove any blood clotting and to apply a clip to the veins. He says things are stable for now, the bleeding has stopped, and he has scheduled surgery for tomorrow afternoon.

Since surgery is not scheduled until mid-afternoon the next day, we bide our time with anticipation. At least we are able to talk with Becki this time around, unlike that cold February day in 1976.

Aimee and Steve arrive from St. Louis just as they are wheeling Becki into surgery. Velda picks up Abie after school and brings her down to the hospital. We sit in the waiting room together, anticipating the outcome.

When the surgery is over, the doctor comes out and tells us everything went very well. In addition to cleaning up the clotted blood and clipping the vein with a titanium clip, he removed the old metal clips from the 1976 surgery and replaced them with titanium also. Gee! I always wanted a new shiny titanium bicycle and Becki gets her titanium before I do. I guess she has a better need for it than I do.

BECKI

Oh, man, I feel like I'm waking up with the hangover from hell. My head feels like concrete, and I feel like every ounce of energy has been drained from my body. It must be early morning because I can just see the sunlight creeping through the window. The nurse comes in and brings me a straw and glass of water.

"Rest," she says, "Denny is here with you and the rest of your family is right outside."

I whisper, "Okay," because I can't move anything else very well, and I close my eyes for a little while. I smile to myself because I am able to give her the answer that was in my head. That's a very good sign.

When I wake up, I see Denny dozing in the chair next to me. He looks a wreck, poor guy. "Denny," I whisper.

Boom Again!

DENNY

She's awake, and she said my name! I feel a heavy weight leave my chest. I knew she would make it through this, but part of me is still afraid that she will get lost inside herself again and that she won't be able to speak and her memories will be robbed from her. Again. But she says my name, and her eyes look clear. I lean over to kiss her. "I told you you'd be okay."

She smiles back at me and slowly mouths the words, "I should listen to you mo-ore of-ten."

BECKI

Abie opens the door and peeks in hesitantly, like a little child unsure of herself. I see her stop at the door and look at me, then she turns around as if she is going to leave. I see her big sister talking to her—I don't know if she is consoling her or reprimanding her. "Come, Abie." I tell her and put out my hand. She walks in slowly and looks at me for the first time since the surgery.

"Mom," she cries and puts her hands to her face like she's witnessing a terrible accident.

I don't think how I must look to her, my head wrapped up like a mummy and hooked up to tubes. "Abie, come here." My words are labored and slow, but I am able to put short sentences together. Tears are streaming down Abie's face and I just want to hold her and make it all better. I hate that I'm the reason she's so scared. "I am okay."

153

Abie comes to me still crying and presses her face against my hand.

"Abie," I tease her, "no wild parties while I'm gone?"

"No, Mom," Abie smiles. "No wild parties."

THE TRIP HOME

BECKI

As I leave the hospital and head home with Denny, I know I have a lot to work on. My speech is slow and slurred and I can't say all the words that are in my head. But, like last time, I will put the puzzle pieces back in place. I know I could've died, but I didn't. And I know death will probably take me with another aneurysm, but not today. Death can go take a hike for now because I'm not ready to go yet.

Denny turns the radio on to Light 93 and I hum along with the music. It's a perfect morning. The sun is breaking through the clouds, promising not to leave. Our family is waiting for us at home, and Denny is next to me. Just like always.

As we get closer to home, *Colour My World* starts playing on the radio. Denny and I exchange looks and smile. What were the chances? There's a gas station coming up, and Denny pulls in. He has a devilish grin on his face as he rushes out of the car and opens my door.

"May I have this dance?"

"Here?" I ask in disbelief.

He nods and takes my hand, gently lifting me out of the car.

We must look such a sight as we slowly sway back and forth, but we don't care. After all, it is our song.

Boom Again!

Words cannot describe how I feel at this moment, and when I look up at Denny, I see all the struggles we've overcome. I see our children laughing and calling things *hernzebekana* with me just so I wouldn't feel badly about my memory loss. I see my daughters reading to me and my husband walking with me, encouraging me not to give up. I see a life worth living.

I say a little prayer and thank God for this day, this hour, and this minute. I know how lucky I am. I realize that moments like these, good and bad, define my life—stringing it together to make a beautiful delicate chain—one that will not end today.

EPILOGUE
(STILL ON THE JOURNEY)
[WRITTEN BY DENNY & BECKI]

BECKI

The focus of my story has been the challenges on the road to recovery from my 1976 stroke, up to my 1998 stroke. However, because it has been more than twenty years since my 1998 stroke, I feel it important to provide a brief synopsis of my continued journey since then.

Recovery from my October 1998 stroke was quicker than the 1976 stroke because the damage was less severe. I took speech therapy from February to June 1999, primarily to learn tricks and techniques to work around my aphasia and also some apraxia of speech (difficulty with motor coordination of speech). I was able to return to work at the school part-time in January, 1999, and continued back, full-time, in the fall of 1999.

In mid-1999, I started experiencing recurrent headaches, not severe but very annoying. My neurosurgeon referred me to a neurologist and we began trying different medications to help with the headaches but also monitoring and changing, as necessary, my seizure medication. For the most part, the headaches improved, but we continued working with the seizure medications.

In summer 2000, Dawn and I started writing this book. In August 2000, a local magazine, *Northshore Lifestyle*, interviewed me and my speech therapist and published an article about my stroke recovery journey and about the book.

During the 2001-2002 school year, things at work became more difficult for me. I experienced a few episodes that might have been mini-seizures (but not the grand mal type). EEG tests showed mini-seizure activity in the brain so we continued to check my medication levels. In May 2002, I received an Outstanding Special Education Aide (i.e., paraprofessional) award from the Wisconsin Council of Administrators and Student Services.

During the spring of 2002, my neurologist and my co-workers encouraged me to consider no longer working, in a polite but somewhat adamant manner. This was a very difficult and emotional decision for me. I knew that it was becoming more difficult for me to make it through the school day, but part of what helped me deal with my stroke recoveries has been a stubborn, "I can do it!" attitude. (Denny agrees with the "stubborn" part of that!) I stopped working in June 2002. Not really a chosen retirement, but rather a medically forced retirement.

In fall 2002, I started volunteering at the hospital where Deb and I took our students for vocational training when I worked at the high school. They allowed me to continue to assist with the same training program, but as a hospital volunteer. I only went in for a couple hours in the early afternoon, but that time helped me transition into no longer being a working woman. I continued volunteering until 2015, when Deb also stopped working in the program.

From December 2002 through February 2003, I again took speech therapy, primarily to help me learn more tricks and techniques to work around my aphasia and apraxia. My speech therapist knew me before I started therapy because she worked at the same hospital where I was volunteering and I would occasionally strike up a conversation with her. She commented after our first meeting that, based on our previous interactions with each other on an informal basis, she was a bit surprised at the level of my communicative disability based on standardized testing. I told her I have spent more than 25 years learning to compensate for my disability (and continue to learn to compensate as additional challenges are provided) so I should be pretty good at it. Essentially, I told her I have learned how to bullshit to make people think I understand what they are saying at times, but I presume I couldn't trick the standardized tests.

In April 2003, I was invited to speak at an annual fundraising dinner at Madonna Rehabilitation Hospital in Lincoln, Nebraska. I spoke about my continuing recovery journey to that point in time. It was a wonderful experience as I was able to get together again with my favorite nun and my speech pathologist from Madonna in the early 1980s. I had not seen either of them for so many years, so it was very special to see them again. In May 2003, I spoke about my stroke recovery journey at the Christian Women's Conference at Valparaiso University, my alma mater.

Other significant happenings since my 1998 stroke are the marriage of our youngest daughter, Abie, in 2006 and the births of our eight grandchildren, between 2000 and 2013. These events are no different or more significant than what anyone else experiences, but they are especially important to me—because Abie is the miracle child we thought we would not be able to have after my first stroke, and I would never have felt the joys of grandchildren if I had not survived the first stroke. Aimee also received her master's degree in speech pathology during this time, a career she chose mostly based on her experience at an early age helping her mother learn how to read better.

With respect to my grandchildren, they have had the unique experience of learning why Grandma Lawton cannot read books to them the same way Mommy, Daddy, Grandpa Lawton, or their other grandparents can. But I can make up one mean and interesting story for them at bedtime. And they all love to feel the "dent" in Grandma's head or make fun of me when they ask me to try to say *Cracker Barrel*. Isn't that grandparent abuse? And they also have learned about my "crazy pills."

I continue to find ways to keep busy at home. Somewhat paradoxically, part of my day gets filled up doing routine things, since it takes me much longer to do many things than most other people. My particular joy is cooking and trying different recipes (Denny says I have enough cookbooks to cook a different meal every day for our next three generations of descendants.) It takes me some time to read through the recipes and then occasionally I forget one of the ingredients (I won't comment on the three tries it took to make a new fudge recipe one Christmas).

I have been able to change my anti-seizure medications from the two I was on for more than 30 years and a third that we added after my 1998 hemorrhage. Two of the medications had potential side effects that ironically can affect my word-finding ability (just what I need) and thinning of bone mass, which I also do not need as I head into my senior years. I am now on only one anti-seizure medication and it does not have those side effects.

I have two final points to make about my experience as an aphasic stroke survivor. One is my desire for more people—including those in the medical profession—to understand the plight of stroke patients who suffer aphasia. We are not stupid or dumb people. Many of us are very intelligent people who just have a short circuit in our communication wiring. Please be patient with us!

160

Epilogue—Still on the Journey

My second point is the importance of my (our) faith in God. I am convinced that my life would have been significantly different if we did not have our faith in the Lord Jesus Christ to guide us through the challenging times.

And I am so very thankful for the support and guidance of our parents, our families, and our many friends and caregivers throughout the last 46 years.

Addendum

A MOTHER'S HEARTACHE— RECOLLECTIONS FROM VELDA MILLER

Below are thoughts that Becki's mother, Velda, provided Dawn and Becki for the book. Velda's manuscript is provided verbatim, based on six hand-written, legal-sized pages. Although some of these recollections are included in the book, we thought these very heartfelt words directly from Velda deserved their own memorializing.

It was a very cold, early Sunday morning. Cal had attended 8 o'clock church and I had just been seated for the late service. The usher came to me and said I had a telephone call. It was Cal, telling me Denny had called. He said something had happened to Becki. They were in the E.R. Becki was not conscious and was having seizures but they didn't know why. He would call back when he knew more. I went home to wait for the call.

I am a nurse so we decided to call the hospital to see if we could learn something from Becki's doctor. They would not give us any information. Then we called the surgeon in Elgin who had removed Becki's gall bladder just a month earlier. He talked to the doctors and was told she apparently was bleeding in the brain but didn't know what from. A neuro-man was to see her.

163

We could not wait any longer so we called Denny and said we were on the way up. Meanwhile we had notified our daughter Gretchen and our son Jim. We quickly packed a few clothes and left.

When we got to Milwaukee, we found Denny in the ICU. Becki was so sick and unstable they were afraid to do further tests. Toward evening, her condition was even more unstable so they had decided to do testing anyway. Poor Den said he had been signing papers all day. After the tests, they said she had to go to surgery to stop the hemorrhage. More papers to sign.

It took many hours of waiting. Finally, the surgeon came and said he had done all he could. The outcome was up to God, and that we should all pray. Of course, we had been doing so all day. Gretchen and her husband came while Becki was in surgery.

After a couple of rough days, we felt she was maybe doing better. Then she started a high temp elevation. Her lungs had thickened and it was difficult to get oxygen into her even with the ventilator. I am not sure how long it went on with her packed in ice—it seemed like forever. We got much better at converting centigrade to Fahrenheit as all her monitors were in centigrade.

Many days went by and she gradually improved. They thought she'd be able to have her G-Tube out. In fact, she reached up and pulled it out herself. Denny and I had worked out a schedule so we could spend time at the hospital. Cal had to go home to work but came up every day off. Early morning, I would go to help Becki with her breakfast and give her a bath.

When Den had to go to school, a friend took care of Aimee until I got home. Den went during his lunch hour. Then Aimee was dropped off with another friend when I went up for suppertime. When I got home, Denny would spend his evening at the hospital and then continue studying when he got home. Working on his masters, caring for a baby and caring for a sick wife was an awful load for a 24-year-old man.

The hospital stay lasted two months. During that time, Becki had many problems. Her right side was paralyzed and she was not able to talk. The damage to the brain was on the left side where the speech center is located. Gradually, the right side improved and she was able to walk with help.

She had a problem eating. She had no appetite and vomited all she did eat. They decided it was from residual swelling in the head and started medications for that.

She was still unable to talk so we used sign language to communicate. She made sounds of a chicken when that was what she wanted. One day she drew a chicken leg to let me know that was what she wanted. One thing she liked—she ate the hospital out of sherbet. Every one of the nurses knew to have some on hand.

A vivid memory of a stormy night will always be with me. The hospital was on Lake Michigan—we could see it from Becki's room. She was not doing well with one setback after another. I was waiting for Denny to come with Aimee. We liked for her to visit so Becki would know she was OK. Looking out at the lake during the storm, I could see large waves coming onto shore. There was rain, snow and sleet. I decided that if God could control anything as big as Lake Michigan, I was sure he could and would help Becki.

After two months, we moved back to the little apartment. Becki did very little but sit and watch T.V. There was so little she could remember to do. Her first tub bath one of many heartaches, as I discovered more problems she had. She had no idea what to do to take a bath but caught on after some "lessons."

One day, I saw her in the kitchen. She had bread and butter out but was just standing there. She was saying a few words and got out "hungry." We had a lesson on making a sandwich. When Denny's friend from college visited, we had dinner. Becki was really trying to be her old self. One mistake. When the butter was passed, she put it on her salad instead of her bread. Each of these and many more events were heartbreaking as we found out what she could not do.

After three months, I decided I had to go home to Elgin. Denny did not really want us to go because I had to take Becki and Aimee with me. I explained I was homesick and felt I should go home to my husband. Denny gave up the apartment, stored their furniture and stayed with a friend while he finished school and wrote his thesis. He came to Elgin on weekends and later went on a field trip—part of his master's program.

Along with loss of speech, we found Becki could not read or write. She had a life-long friend who was a speech pathologist, who came twice a week all summer and helped so much to gain much of her speech back.

At the end of six months, I went back to work. Becki had Aimee's care for the first time. Cal was home for breakfast and lunch to help out. She still did no cooking, cleaning or laundry. I did basic care for Aimee like bathing in the evening.

Denny was looking for work and found it in Nebraska. What a long way away. When we helped them move, Cal and I had so many questions about care for both the girls. Needless to say, I had become very attached to Aimee after caring for her over eight months. When we left them, I thought my heart would break. We wondered how Den was going to care for them and do his work.

The people there were wonderful—especially the minister and his wife and a close neighbor. We went out as often as we could which was only a couple times a year. Each time we could see improvement in Becki. She and Aimee practiced talking together and worked on big words.

Later they moved to Lincoln, Nebraska, where Den worked at the university. Becki started at a rehab center. They were wonderful and lots of help. Abie was born 5 years after Aimee.

We were so happy when they moved back to Milwaukee. We were able to see them more and then eventually life was quite normal. The girls did very well in school. Becki got work at the school working with special-ed kids. The family had friends and had a good social life. All was well.

Then October 12th, 1998, we got another early a.m. call. We couldn't believe what Denny was saying. Becki was back in the ICU with another hemorrhage. We are so thankful it was not nearly as severe as the first time. Again, we packed a few things and went up. Again, Gretchen came in time for the surgery. We had been through all of this before but it does not keep us from being so afraid. Becki and family are all working very hard to regain all that she had accomplished, including giving Abie a high school graduation party and teaching her special education children.

I don't know how I can put on paper the heartache her dad and I have had. We are just thankful for all that Denny and good friends have done for her.

PHOTO GALLERY

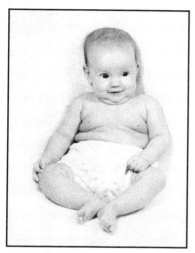

Becki, about 6 months
(little did anyone know she had an
AVM growing inside her head).

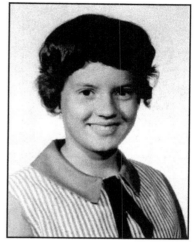

Becki in 6th grade
(likely when she had her first
AVM bleed).

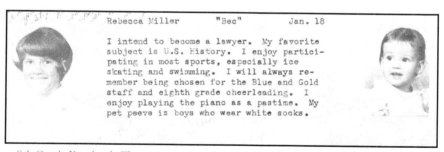

Rebecca Miller   "Bec"   Jan. 18

I intend to become a lawyer. My favorite
subject is U.S. History. I enjoy partici-
pating in most sports, especially ice
skating and swimming. I will always remember being chosen for the Blue and Gold
staff and eighth grade cheerleading. I
enjoy playing the piano as a pastime. My
pet peeve is boys who wear white socks.

8th Grade Yearbook. Things were already getting harder for Becki. Her teachers and
counselors noticed it but no one tied it back to the 6th-grade incident.
Her aspiration was to be a lawyer.

Hernzebekana! Her Language of Love

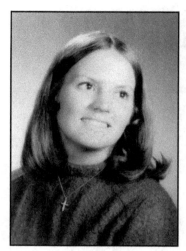

1970—High School Graduation. Becki still read a lot of books but retention was probably already affected.

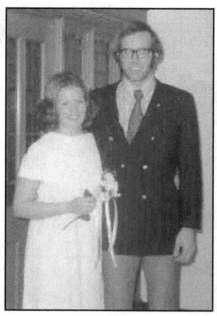

Fall 1971—Denny and Becki started dating as sophomores at Valparaiso University.

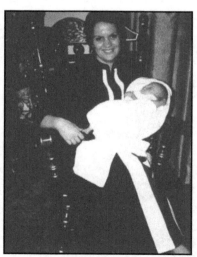

November 1975—Aimee was born. It was the beginning of a busy three months.

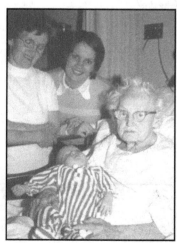

January 1976—Four generations with Grandma Van. Hours later, the family drove back to Elgin in the middle of the night for Becki's gall bladder surgery.

Photo Gallery

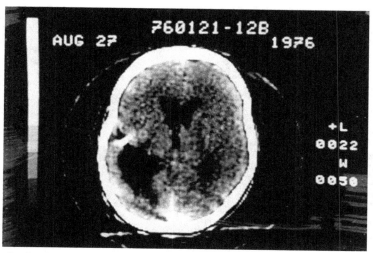

Becki's brain on February 1, 1976. This is the CAT scan performed about seven months later, one of the first CAT scans done in the Milwaukee area. The shiny feature in the middle of the left side is a metal clip that blocks off the main artery feeding the AVM.

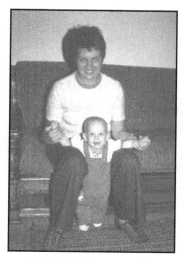

April 1976—Just out of the hospital, back in Elgin with Mom and Dad.

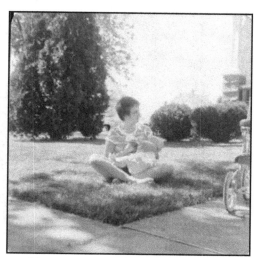

May 1976—Learning to be a mom again.

Hernzebekana! Her Language of Love

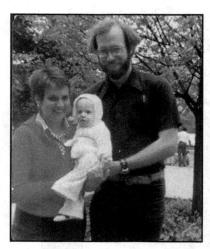

Summer 1976—Becki and Denny just learned they were moving to Nebraska.

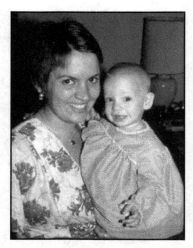

August 1976—Aimee at 9 months and Becki 6 months post-stroke.

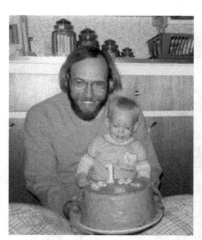

November 1976—Aimee's first birthday and Becki's first post-stroke cake baking.

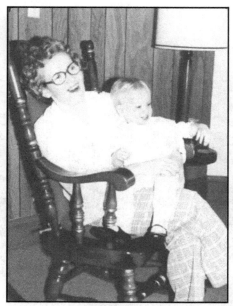

Grandma Velda enjoying Aimee. Velda helped take care of her granddaughter for several months during Becki's recovery.

Photo Gallery

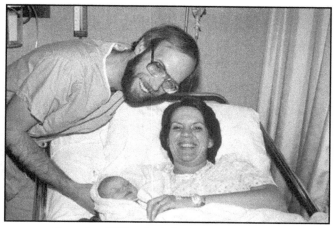

November 1980—Abie's birth. Their "miracle."

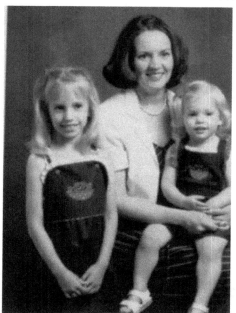

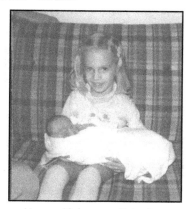

Aimee with her new little sister.

*Early 1980s—Becki and the girls,
trying to live a normal life—sort of.*

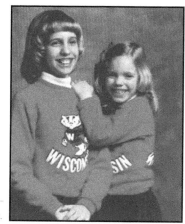

*November 1986—
Back n Wisconsin.*

Hernzebekana! Her Language of Love

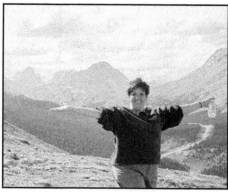

Summer 1998—Denny and Becki's 25th anniversary. After hiking up Parker Ridge Trail in the Canadian Rockies.

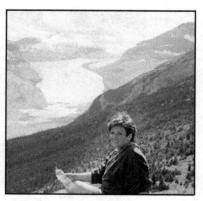

The prize at the top of Parker Ridge: the Saskatchewan Glacier.

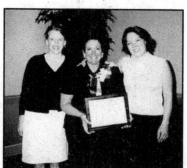

May 2020—Becki receiving the Outstanding Special Education Aide Award with her co-teachers. Dawn (in white blouse) is standing next to her.

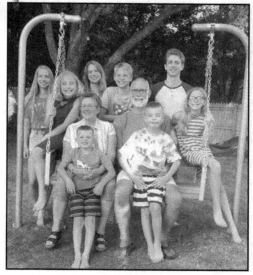

Spring 2020—Becki and Denny with their eight grandchildren.

RESOURCES

Below is a list of some organizations that provide resources related to stroke and aphasia. There also may be other relevant organizations not listed below. Our listing of these organizations is not a specific endorsement from us, nor does it imply an endorsement by them of this book.

- National Aphasia Association (aphasia.org)
- Aphasia Recovery Connection (aphasiarecoveryconnection.org)
- Brain Buddy (brainbuddy.org)
- Aphasia Hope Foundation (aphasiahope.org)
- American Stroke Association - A Division of the American Heart Association (stroke.org)
- American Stroke Foundation (americanstroke.org)
- Brain Injury Association (biausa.org)
- Brain Aneurysm Foundation (bafound.org)

Please also visit our website:
www.HerLanguageOfLove.com

Hernzebekana! Her Language of Love

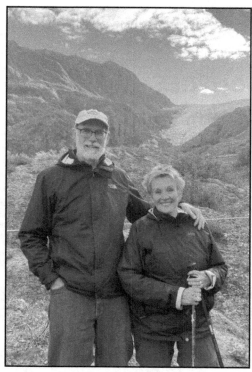

Denny and Becki hiking at Exit Glacier near Seward, Alaska (September 2022).

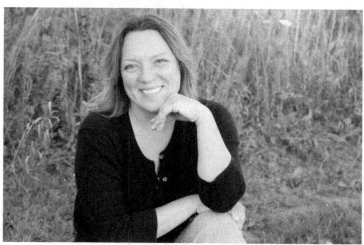

Dawn Rosewitz

ABOUT THE AUTHORS

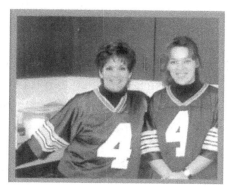

Becki and Dawn in Packers jerseys during homecoming week—three days before the October 1998 stroke.

BECKI

In 1974, Rebecca (Becki) Lawton completed her English degree from Valparaiso University. Then, on February 1, 1976, three months after the birth of her first daughter, she suffered a severe hemorrhagic stroke: a ruptured arteriovenous malformation (AVM). With professional and family help, she learned to live with her aphasia. Her second daughter was born in November, 1980. Eight years later, Becki was able to work as a special education paraprofessional, helping children whose challenges she understood, first hand. In 1998, however, she suffered another, less severe, hemorrhagic stroke and was forced to stop working. Today, Becki and her husband, Denny, are enjoying retirement and their eight grandkids. Becki continues to navigate challenges with her aphasia.

DAWN

Dawn Rosewitz has been a special education teacher for almost 30 years. Her students inspired her to create *The Land of Ican* series to help them understand they can accomplish many things, just in their own unique ways! (Available on Amazon.com.) It was published by Roger Hammer, *A Place in the Woods*. She has also contributed articles to educational magazines. Later, when she began working with Becki Lawton, they struck up a friendship and a two-year partnership that culminated in this book. When she's not teaching or enjoying time with her family, she's working on her next story!